SURE FOOTING

A Sports Podiatrist's Perspective on Running- and Exercise-Related Injuries

Perry H. Julien, DPM

Atlanta Foot and Ankle Center
5600 Roswell Road
Suite 390 East
Atlanta, GA 30342
(404) 255–9131

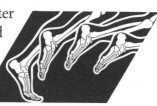

Credits

EDITING, DESIGN, LAYOUT, AND PRODUCTION: Jan and Joe Seeley
FRONT COVER PHOTO: Chris Hamilton
BACK COVER PHOTO: Rod Kaye
MEDICAL ILLUSTRATIONS: James Zelichowski, DPM
DEDICATION PAGE CARTOON: Michael Hughes
MANUSCRIPT PREPARATION: Ivey S. Davis

Special thanks

◢ to my staff at the Atlanta Foot and Ankle Center for their support, input, patience, (and tolerance);

◢ to Christine Donnelly, Robin Myers, and Laura Weldon for editing the original articles for *Atlanta Sports and Fitness Magazine*; and

◢ to Jan and Joe Seeley, who made the idea for this book a reality.

To Lisa and Monika…
For being there every step of the way.

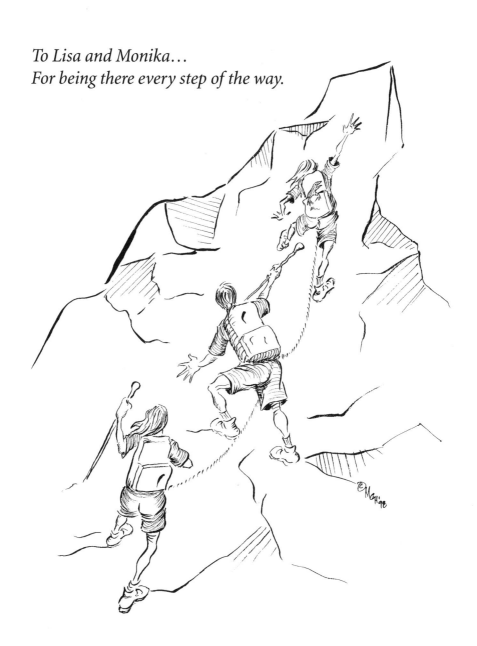

Contents

Preface

SPORTS MEDICINE IS AS MUCH A PHILOSOPHY AS IT IS A SPECIALTY. Although the motivation may be different, the desire for the weekend athlete to stay active is often as great as the Olympian training for international competition. The more insight and understanding individuals have of their injury, the greater role they can then play in their treatment and ultimate return to full activity.

The idea for *Sure Footing* began as a desire to provide our Atlanta Foot and Ankle Center patients with written information on the lower extremity problems that brought them to our office for treatment. My goal was to translate the information available in medical textbooks to a format that would be more understandable but still contain the same level of material, for those who wanted to take an active role in the recognition, treatment, and prevention of their injuries. *Sure Footing* resulted from a collection of these articles and other writings combined with photographs and illustrations to further explain topics that might not be clear to individuals who do not have a medical background.

My sports medicine knowledge has not come just from books. I have been fortunate to be surrounded by and to learn from many individuals who have a passion for treating active people. Too numerous to mention by name, this list includes physicians, podiatrists, physiologists, physical therapists, athletic trainers, chiropractors, massage therapists, and coaches. The greatest lessons I have learned, however, have come from the athletes and active people that I have had the privilege to examine and treat. The knowledge gathered from opportunities such as working with David E. Martin, PhD, and the USATF Elite Athlete Project and being a part of the Olympic Medical Support Group during the 1996 Summer Olympic Games have also furthered my understanding of the spectrum of available medical management for active individuals at all levels. The concepts we use to help elite-level competitors who push beyond the extremes of human performance can be applied to those whose training goals are much less intense.

I hope *Sure Footing* provides a valuable resource for you, to help you understand better the implications of normal and abnormal function of the lower extremities, to serve as a starting point for prevention and self-treatment, and to guide you when medical intervention becomes necessary.

Perry H. Julien, DPM
May 1998

If the Shoe Fits
Selecting an Athletic Shoe

FOR HEALTH-CONSCIENCE INDIVIDUALS, SELECTING PROPER athletic shoes is extremely important. Many of the common overuse injuries seen by sports medicine physicians can be attributed directly or indirectly to improper shoes. Choosing appropriate footwear will not only help prevent injuries but will also let you participate to the best of your ability.

To choose the correct shoes, you should consider the activity they will be used for, your foot type and biomechanics, and any existing foot problems. Knowing something about shoe anatomy and foot function will then help you make an educated decision regarding the best shoe for you.

Anatomy of an Athletic Shoe

Athletic shoes, especially those used for running or walking, typically emphasize either motion control (stability) or shock absorption (cushioning) in their design. Unfortunately, these two functions often contradict each other. Generally speaking, a softer, cushioned shoe offers less support and stability than a firmer shoe.

Many components of an athletic shoe combine to determine the way it functions. When selecting a shoe, you should consider the toe box, midsole, counter, and last (Figures 1.1 and 1.2).

The **toe box** is the front part of the upper of a shoe, where the toes lie. The width and height of the toe box vary among brands and models. The size of the toe box is particularly important for people with bunions, hammertoes, and other "fit" problems related to the front part of their feet. These conditions can be irritated by toe boxes that are too small.

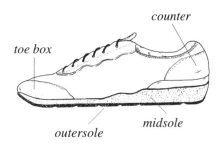

Figure 1.1 Anatomy of an athletic shoe

The **midsole** of a shoe, usually made of ethylene vinyl acetate (EVA) or polyurethane, provides cushioning and shock absorption for the body. It is in this portion of the shoe that many of the shock absorbing inserts such as air and gel are incorporated.

The **counter** of the shoe wraps around the back of the heel and provides motion control and stability for the foot.

The **last** is the form around which the shoe is built (Figure 1.2). This shape determines many of the functional characteristics of the shoe and is often classified as being straight, semicurved, or curved.

A straight-lasted shoe is filled in on the inside or medial part of the shoe, which increases its stability and generally allows it to fit a flat arch better.

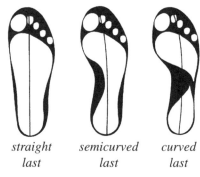

straight last   semicurved last   curved last

Figure 1.2 Shoe last shapes

A semicurved last, designed for the average foot, has a small curve on the inside and is the best last shape for most fitness-minded individuals. Most court shoes and aerobic shoes are built on semicurved lasts, as are most running and walking shoes. The curvature of a semicurved last depends on the specific brand and model of the shoe.

Finally, a shoe built on a curved last is designed for those with higher than normal arches and for those who underpronate. In addition to the curve in these shoes, the outside or lateral portion is wider, which provides forefoot stability for underpronation. This type of shoe is usually reserved for faster runners. Faster runners are often midfoot strikers, which means they land on the front part of their feet. Midfoot strikers with no previous history of injuries tend to run better in shoes built on a semicurved or curved last. Many midfoot strikers also require shoes with increased cushioning in the forefoot to absorb some of the ground forces.

Despite all the advances in shoe design and material over the last several years, athletic shoes do not last forever. Depending on your weight, your foot type, and the activities that the shoes are used for, you should expect a shoe to last between 300 and 500 walking or jogging miles or three to five months. Although a shoe may not look worn-out, often the midsole or counter will have begun to break down, which decreases the shoe's cushioning and support and affects the function of the shoe.

Foot Type

Foot type is often categorized by arch height. The arch of the foot is formed by bones and is supported by muscles, tendons, and ligaments. Arches may be considered high (cavus), moderate, or low (planus). Your arch height should always be evaluated when you are standing with full weight on your feet, because a flexible foot may appear to have a higher arch when there is no pressure placed on it. High-arched feet have smaller weight-bearing areas when they contact the ground and also tend to be more rigid, resulting in greater stress being transmitted to the foot and leg. A runner with a high arch may want to select a shoe that provides greater cushioning and shock absorption to make up for the lack of normal shock-reducing capabilities in this foot type. A high-arched foot will also tend to function better in a semicurve- or curve-lasted shoe.

If you have a low-arched foot, it is generally a flexible foot that may be subject to excessive motion when you walk or run. This motion may lead to overuse injuries. In a flexible, low-arched foot, motion control and stability are of prime importance when you select an athletic shoe. Often a straight- or mild semicurve-lasted shoe will be most appropriate. If you are a significant overpronator, you may need orthotics to control the foot properly.

Foot Biomechanics

Pronation is a foot motion that occurs normally when the heel strikes the ground to help the body absorb the impact. This motion appears as a flattening of the arch or a rolling in of the foot.

Pronation is a problem only when it becomes excessive. Overpronation can be the result of inherited foot structure, muscle or tendon imbalances, leg length differences, or other biomechanical irregularities. A foot that overpronates is often considered an unstable foot; and while it is usually good at absorbing shock, it may not be stable enough to prevent certain injuries. In these circumstances, a shoe model that incorporates motion-control characteristics will be more beneficial than one with extra cushioning. In some cases, the control afforded by a shoe is not enough, and custom orthotics may be required to correct this excessive motion. Even with orthotics, however, proper shoe selection is essential if you're going to get the right amount of motion control.

Supination is the opposite of pronation. It occurs normally right after heel strike to help the foot become a rigid lever to propel off of. Oversupination is very rare. What is more common is underpronation, which can occur with a rigid, high-arched foot. A foot that underpronates is not able to absorb impact very well, which can lead to stress fractures, heel pain, knee pain, and other injuries. A foot that underpronates needs a shoe capable of absorbing shock well. Motion control is usually not very important in this type of foot; however, in some cases orthotics can distribute pressure and support this foot type.

Many feet fit in between these two extremes, and shoe companies have responded to this need by designing more versatile shoes that provide both cushioning and the necessary amount of motion control in one model.

Evaluating over- and underpronation by watching someone walk or run can be difficult for the untrained observer. This judgment should be left to your physician, athletic shoe fitter, or coach. You can be misled by improperly evaluating wear patterns on the bottom of athletic shoes. Normal foot strike occurs on the outside portion of the heel area, where most shoes typically exhibit excessive wear. This pattern is normal. On the other hand, a counter that bends inward is usually a reliable sign that overpronation is taking place. The continued improvements in athletic shoe material will typically make it difficult to determine subtle biomechanical abnormalities unless the shoe itself is significantly broken down or the biomechanical problem is severe.

Your weight is also important when you are selecting a shoe based on foot biomechanics. An active person who weighs around 150 pounds and overpronates may not require as much stability from a specific shoe model as a heavier individual with a similar foot type. Although the actual biomechanical function of the foot may be similar, a shoe that offers a high degree of motion control may be too firm for a lighter active person and could result in overuse injuries.

Existing Foot Problems

You also have to consider existing foot problems when you are selecting an athletic shoe. A history of fitness-related injuries may be the result of abnormal foot biomechanics that can be controlled with proper athletic shoes, or may be an indication that your athletic shoes are not correct for your needs. If you have bony deformities such as bunions, hammertoes, and bone spurs, you may have to select a shoe with a wide or high toe box or make sure the upper of the shoe does not irritate any painful areas on the foot. If a specific shoe model seems to make an existing injury worse, that model should be evaluated with respect to your foot type to make certain it is not aggravating the injury.

Sport-Specific Use

You must also consider the type of activity you will use the shoe for. Ideally, athletic shoes should be worn only for the sport for which they were designed. Shoes for sports that require side-to-side motion, such as tennis and racquetball, may have more support and stability than is needed for running and walking. However, running and walking shoes have characteristics that make them unsuitable for side-to-side sports such as tennis, racquetball, or step aerobics. It can be expensive to use specific shoes for different sports, but the benefits of increased performance and decreased injury risk are well worth the extra investment.

Shoe Fit

The most important consideration in choosing an athletic shoe is fit. If a shoe does not fit correctly and comfortably, it will not function as it was designed to, negating the benefits of any motion control or cushioning it has. The following guidelines will help you when you are trying on different models of shoes that may be appropriate for your needs:

1. When trying on shoes, always use a similar weight sock and any additional devices such as orthotics that you plan to wear with the shoes.
2. Leave at least ¼ inch (one finger's width) between your longest toe and the end of the shoe. The counter of the shoe should be snug enough that the heel does not slide up and down excessively.
3. Take into consideration that feet tend to swell when you have been standing or exercising, and this could affect the proper sizing of the shoe. Therefore, it is better to shop for shoes later in the day.
4. Make sure you try on both shoes fully laced and walk or run in the store to assure comfort and fit. It is often a good idea to wear the shoes at home on a carpeted or hardwood floor for a few hours prior to taking the shoes on the road. Do not rely too much on breaking in the shoe to provide comfort.

Selecting a proper athletic shoe is both an art and a science. Fortunately, most athletic shoe stores employ people who have a knowledge of the factors that go into choosing the "right" shoes. In more difficult fitting situations, you may want to work with a sports podiatrist to help select the best shoes for your foot type and function. By understanding basic lower extremity biomechanics and shoe design, you should be able to narrow down your choices to a few models and then let comfort and fit be your guide. ◢

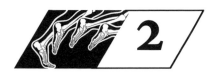

Stretching
The Importance of
Lower Extremity Flexibility

FLEXIBILITY IS OFTEN ACKNOWLEDGED AS AN IMPORTANT PART OF injury prevention, yet much controversy exists regarding overstretching and understretching.

Muscles should be flexible enough to allow the joints they control to function through their normal range of motion. If this motion is restricted, the muscle or tendon may stretch past its range, thus directly resulting in injuries such as tears or strains.

Although many muscle groups function in lower extremity movement, adequate flexibility of the calf muscles is particularly important in preventing injuries of the foot and leg.

The Calf Muscles
The calf muscles are the strongest muscles of the lower leg. They consist of the gastrocnemius and soleus muscles and are joined to the heel bone (calcaneus) by the Achilles tendon. The calf muscles assist in moving the foot and ankle downward (plantarflexion), which helps propel the body forward. If this area lacks flexibility, an injury such as a tear or strain of the calf muscles or Achilles tendon may result.

The foot and leg may also compensate for the restricted range of motion due to calf tightness by pronating the feet excessively. While this condition may not directly cause injury, it can indirectly result in problems. Pronation, which appears as a flattening of the arch, causes the joints of the foot to become more flexible so they can absorb impact when the foot hits the ground. Overpronation can make the foot unstable and lead to injuries such as plantar fasciitis, Achilles tendonitis, shin pain, and other overuse injuries.

Many of our daily activities can result in calf tightness. Standing and walking in high-heeled shoes will shorten the calf muscles, as will sitting for long periods of time. When we sleep, our feet usually point downward, and blankets can accentuate this position by applying a small amount of pressure to the top of the foot. All these activities can result in decreased motion at the ankle joint over time. Dehydration can also play a role in calf inflexibility due to the large amount of water contained in the calf muscles.

The Goal of Stretching

The goal of proper stretching is to achieve enough flexibility that the joints acted on by specific muscles can function within their normal range of motion. Consistency with stretching is much more important than intensity in reaching this goal. A hard stretch will only tear muscles and tendons and may even cause the tendon to reflexively shorten. By stretching frequently and gradually, you allow your muscles to adapt slowly to the lengthened position, increasing flexibility.

The following stretch makes the calf muscles more flexible:

1. Place the leg you are stretching behind you with the heel on the ground and the foot facing straight ahead (Figure 2.1).
2. Avoid flattening the arch; you may need to roll the foot outward slightly to accomplish this (Figure 2.2).
3. Lean forward until you feel a mild pull in the calf muscle. You should not feel any significant stretch in the Achilles tendon area. If this is painful, you are probably stretching too hard.

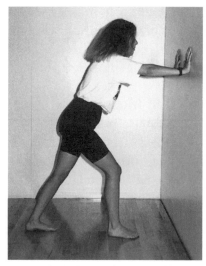

Figure 2.1: Calf muscle stretch

PERRY H. JULIEN, DPM

4. Hold this stretch for 10 seconds and repeat three times with each leg.

You can repeat this stretch several times throughout the day. Be careful not to overstretch; you may have to place your foot different distances from the wall based on your current level of flexibility.

By keeping your knee straight, you will stretch the gastrocnemius muscle, which is closer to your knee. In most instances, this muscle will be less flexible than the soleus. To isolate the soleus, bend your knee slightly when executing the stretch, but be careful not to put stress on the Achilles tendon.

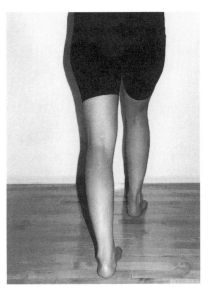

Figure 2.2: Proper foot position for stretching the calf muscles

There are also several devices that you can use to place your foot and leg in an optimal position to achieve a satisfactory stretch. One such device, a dorsiflexion splint (Figure 2.3) that is worn while you sleep, places a mild stretch on the calf muscles. It is sometimes used to treat conditions such as plantar fasciitis and Achilles tendonitis.

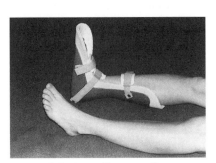

Figure 2.3: Dorsiflexion splint

Regardless of the stretching methods you choose, consistency and patience are essential in developing adequate flexibility. Aggressive overstretching can actually lead to the development of other injuries.

Stretching exercises are often incorporated into rehabilitation programs for many overuse injuries. By establishing a regular program of lower extremity stretching, you can often prevent these injuries from developing, allowing yourself to continue with your fitness goals. ◢

3

So What If I Pronate?

INCREASED PARTICIPATION IN SPORTS ACTIVITIES IN ALL AGE GROUPS has made people more aware of health and fitness issues. Magazines and newspapers regularly print articles on diet, nutrition, training, and injuries. Fitness-oriented individuals are constantly seeking ways to improve their performance while staying healthy and injury-free.

One sports medicine topic that receives a great deal of attention, especially with runners and walkers, is overpronation. If you listened in on a group of runners talking about their aches and pains, you would certainly hear them discussing overpronation at some point. Unfortunately, despite all the information available about foot biomechanics, very few people understand what actually takes place from the time the foot hits the ground until it pushes off (the gait cycle) and how it can lead to injuries. Many people would actually be surprised to hear that pronation is a normal part of foot function.

What Is Pronation?

Our lower extremities go through a complex series of movements that propel us forward. One of the most important functions of the foot is to help the body absorb shock when it hits the ground. Depending on the activities in which we participate, our lower extremities experience a force between one-and-a-half to three times our body weight every time our feet hit the ground.

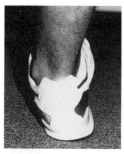

Figure 3.1: Heel strike

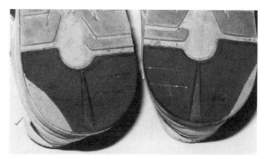

Figure 3.2: Normal sole wear pattern

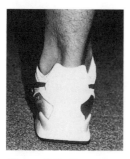

Figure 3.3: Pronation

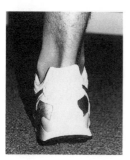

Figure 3.4: Supination

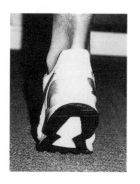

Figure 3.5: Push-off

The foot normally strikes the ground on the outside (lateral) part of the heel (Figure 3.1), which is why our shoes tend to wear on the outside back portion of the heel (Figure 3.2). As soon as the foot hits the ground, the heel rolls inward. This motion — pronation — absorbs shock and gives the appearance that the arch is flattening out (Figure 3.3). This pronation mechanism unlocks the bones in the foot, making it more flexible and reducing the force to the feet, ankles, knees, hips, and back. Once this pronation phase is complete, the foot begins to roll out or supinate slightly (Figure 3.4), creating a more stable and rigid foot position that allows the lower extremity to achieve maximum efficiency when pushing off (Figure 3.5).

Pronation, then, is a normal, necessary biomechanical motion in foot function. However, if the foot pronates too much (see Figure 3.6) or for too long, it will remain unstable, making the lower extremities less supportive of body weight. This can result in heel or arch pain, stress fractures, knee pain, other overuse injuries, and even bunions, hammertoes, and bone spurs.

Pronation also occurs in other sports that do not involve walking or running. When skiers make a turn, pronation helps set an edge so that the ski does not skid; however, overpronation in a ski boot can result in wasted motion, making it more difficult for a skier to begin a turn. This extra effort can also cause greater fatigue for the skier.

Likewise, cyclists can pronate excessively when pedaling. Although there is no impact in cycling, certain lower extremity biomechanical abnormalities in an athlete may actually cause overpronation while the rider pushes down on the pedals. As in skiing, this extra motion decreases efficiency and can cause fatigue. Overpronation can also cause the knee to move inward and can result in knee pain and discomfort.

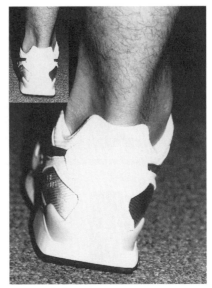

Figure 3.6: Overpronation;
(inset: Normal pronation)

The Causes of Overpronation

Overpronation can result from several causes. Our foot shape is, to a great extent, genetically predetermined. The position of the bones and joints can cause the foot to assume an overpronated position. This condition is sometimes obvious in a child when he begins to walk and can get progressively worse as the child's weight and activity level increase.

Overpronation can also result from biomechanical abnormalities. If part of the foot or leg lacks the normal range of motion necessary for walking or running, another nearby joint may be required to compensate for this lack of motion. For example, tight calf muscles are one of the most common biomechanical problems causing overpronation. The foot needs to bend upwards 5 to 10 degrees at the ankle for normal lower extremity motion to occur. If this motion is unavailable because of calf muscle tightness, the foot will overpronate to make up for this limitation. Stretching the calf muscles properly will reduce these forces acting on the foot and can help prevent lower extremity injuries.

Finally, wearing improper shoes is another cause of overpronation. If a shoe is worn-out or broken down, it cannot function as it was designed. Wearing the wrong type of shoe can also cause overpronation. Sports shoes that have a curved last tend to increase the amount of pronation that occurs in the foot and can cause problems in a foot that is unstable or overpronates.

Many shoes are categorized as motion control shoes, which means that the shoes have a straighter last and more supportive materials on the inner (medial) side of the shoe. These modifications are designed to limit the amount of inward roll, or pronation. They won't completely stop pronation, but they will let this motion occur within "normal" limits. Runners can also use foot-supporting devices called orthotics to control excessive abnormal motion, including overpronation.

Recognizing Overpronation

You can detect overpronation in several ways. You can best observe it by watching someone walk or run from behind. The more the back of the heel rolls in and the arch flattens out, the greater the amount of pronation that is occurring. In an overpronated foot, you may also notice a slight bowing outward of the Achilles tendon. It is more difficult to assess overpronation by examining shoe wear. The outer soles of most athletic shoes are now made from very durable material and do not always reflect the true biomechanics of the person wearing them. Excessive wear on the outside of the heel does not indicate overpronation — that is the normal location of heel strike when you run or walk. The part of the shoe that will reflect excessive pronation is the counter, which is the area that supports and cradles the heel. With excessive pronation, this counter will eventually break down to the inside. This shoe condition is also a sign that the shoe is no longer providing good stability for the foot.

It is often difficult to assess how destructive overpronation can be to the lower extremities. Many world-class athletes overpronate, but these athletes function well in their respective sports with few injuries. Yet, others with less severe overpronation problems experience many overuse injuries that can be linked to this abnormal foot motion, including stress fractures, heel pain, Achilles tendonitis, posterior tibial tendonitis, bunions, and bone spurs.

Pronation occurs in varying degrees every time our feet strike the ground and even in other sports where direct impact is not present. If you feel your feet roll in excessively, and you seem to be plagued with various lower extremity ailments, a thorough biomechanical examination can help determine the extent to which overpronation is contributing to these problems. Your physician can then recommend steps to control this motion to acceptable levels. ◢

4

The Painful Heel

HEEL PAIN CAN AFFECT ALL ACTIVE INDIVIDUALS, FROM RECRE-ational walkers to elite athletes. The heel bone (calcaneus) is a connecting point for several tendons, ligaments, fascia, and muscles. Several nerves also surround the heel on both sides. Given this complex anatomy, it is easy to see why heel pain makes up one of the largest categories of overuse injuries in active people.

In most instances these problems result from overtraining, improper footwear, or some form of biomechanical abnormality such as a rigid, high-arched foot or a flexible, overpronated foot. To treat heel pain effectively, you must first pinpoint the cause so you can take specific steps to alleviate pain and prevent a recurrence. The most common causes of heel pain include plantar fasciitis/calcaneal spur syndrome, heel bursitis, calcaneal stress fractures, and nerve injuries.

Plantar Fasciitis/Heel Spur Syndrome

Plantar fasciitis is the most common form of heel pain in active individuals. Initially, the pain from plantar fasciitis will occur when you take the first few steps after getting out of bed or sitting for a long time. The pain is often described as feeling like a stone bruise and will usually improve after walking for a little while. As this injury becomes more severe, you can feel pain anytime you stand or walk.

Plantar fasciitis is an inflammation of the band of tissue located along the bottom of the foot that extends from the heel bone to the

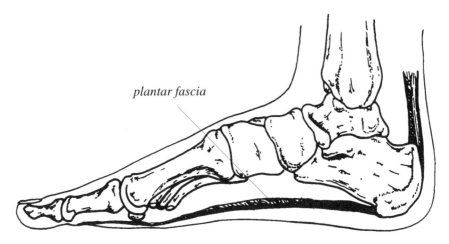

plantar fascia

Figure 4.1: Plantar fascia

base of the toes and supports the arch of the foot (Figure 4.1). This band of tissue is relatively inflexible, and when stressed, it will usually pull from the heel bone, which causes pain. Over time, the constant pulling of the fascia on the heel bone can cause a bone spur to form on the bottom of the heel (Figure 4.2). The presence of a heel spur is usually a good indication that the problem has been present for some time, even if symptoms have only recently developed. The pulling of the fas-

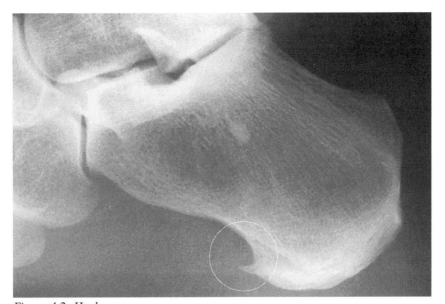

Figure 4.2: Heel spur

cia usually causes the pain; very rarely does the spur itself cause discomfort.

Plantar fasciitis can result from overtraining, contact with hard or irregular surfaces during walking or exercising, and structural or biomechanical abnormalities affecting the foot or leg. These abnormalities include rigid, high-arched feet and overpronation.

A high-arched foot can be predisposed to plantar fasciitis because of the inability of this foot type to absorb shock, which increases stress on the fascia. However, overpronation is a much more common cause of plantar fasciitis due to the stretching of the fascia at its origin as the arch flattens out.

Treating Plantar Fasciitis/Heel Spur Syndrome

Treatment for plantar fasciitis/heel spur syndrome is broken down into two categories: pain reduction and correction of the causative factors. Applying ice for 15 minutes two or three times daily can help reduce pain. This treatment has the advantage of providing an anti-inflammatory effect directly to the heel with little risk of undesirable side effects. Nonsteroidal anti-inflammatories such as ibuprofen can also alleviate discomfort; however, these pills do not solve the problem, and in most cases they provide only temporary relief. Injecting cortisone in the heel is not usually a first-line treatment, but it can be effective when chronic inflammation persists. In general, you shouldn't have more than three cortisone injections in one specific region of the foot because of the effects cortisone can have on the surrounding tissue.

The most important aspect of treating plantar fasciitis/heel spur syndrome is to correct or control the factors that may have led to the injury. The most common cause of plantar fasciitis is a stretching of the fascia itself, which may be directly caused by an overpronated foot or indirectly caused by tightness of the calf muscles.

When the calf muscles are tight, motion in the ankle joint can be restricted, which prevents the ankle from bending up (dorsiflexing) enough for normal walking or running. To compensate for this lack of dorsiflexion, the foot may overpronate, creating excessive pull on the plantar fascia. Other factors that can contribute to overpronation include leg length differences, tight hamstrings, and inherited biomechanical foot structure.

An important component in the long-term treatment of plantar fasciitis is developing adequate flexibility in the calf muscle area. There are many different stretches for this part of the body, and proper technique is essential in achieving good results. In some circumstances, you may use a device called a dorsiflexion splint (Figure 4.3) or night splint to keep the foot in a 90-degree position while you sleep. This can help treat plantar fasciitis as well as other lower extremity overuse injuries.

Although the bottom of the heel is the primary area of discomfort in plantar fasciitis, the actual mechanism causing pain is a stretching of the plantar fascia itself. For this reason heel cups or heel cushions rarely offer significant relief from this condition. The goal of treatment should be to support the plantar fascia to prevent it from pulling excessively. You can often accomplish this by taping or padding the arch or using some form of arch support. If, despite these self-treatment methods, your heel pain persists, your sports medicine physician may recommend orthotics. These orthotics are designed to correct or control abnormal foot structure or biomechanics. Properly prescribed orthotics will allow the bones, muscles, and tendons to function more efficiently, thus taking stress off the fascia and hopefully relieving your symptoms.

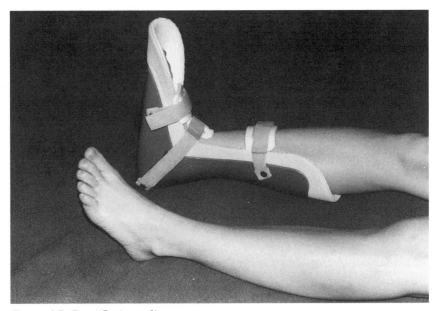

Figure 4.3: Dorsiflexion splint

Most cases of plantar fasciitis/heel spur syndrome will improve with conservative treatment. If your pain persists after you have exhausted conservative care options, surgery may be indicated.

Heel Surgery

Traditionally, surgery for heel spur syndrome and plantar fasciitis required a large open incision to release the fascia and remove the bone spur. More recently, the use of endoscopy has enabled a surgeon to release the fascia without significant trauma to the surrounding tissue. This procedure, known as endoscopic plantar fasciotomy (EPF), is performed by placing two small incisions on each side of the heel where an endoscope is placed. This endoscope allows the surgeon to see the fascia, which is then partially released (Figure 4.4) with a special instrument. The heel spur is not removed, as this is not usually a cause of pain. Although the recovery from EPF is less involved than recovery from open heel spur surgery, it may still take several weeks for full healing to take place. Surgery for plantar fasciitis should only be considered after exhausting all conservative options to resolve your pain.

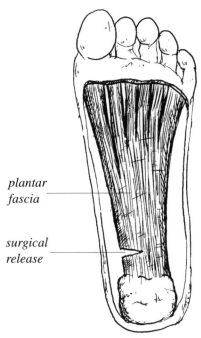

plantar
fascia

surgical
release

Figure 4.4: Surgical release of plantar fascia

To prevent plantar fasciitis, you should be careful to increase your physical activity gradually and pay careful attention to warm-up, cool-down, and appropriate stretching before and after exercise. Be aware of the surfaces on which you exercise, and make sure your athletic shoes fit correctly and are not worn-out. Finally, control any biomechanical abnormalities under the guidance of your sports medicine physician.

Heel Bursitis

A bursa is a fluid-filled sac that provides cushioning in certain parts of the body. The heel has a bursa that lies directly underneath the calcaneus. When subject to stress from overtraining or exercising on hard surfaces without adequate cushion, this bursa can become inflamed. The symptoms of heel bursitis can resemble those of plantar fasciitis, with pain occurring when you first stand in the morning. However, with heel bursitis the pain will usually persist with any weight-bearing activity and can often be felt directly underneath the heel bone.

Treatment for heel bursitis usually includes replacing worn-out athletic shoes, using some type of cushioned footbed inside your shoes, and applying ice to reduce inflammation. If these measures do not resolve the problem, your physician may recommend cortisone injections or orthotics.

Calcaneal Stress Fractures

A stress fracture is a true break in the bone resulting from repetitive, low-grade impact or trauma that eventually weakens the bone to the point of fracture.

The heel bone is subject to a great deal of stress during fitness activities. Studies have shown that our lower extremities undergo forces up to three times our body weight during running, much of which is often directed at the heel bone. Symptoms of a stress fracture can also mimic plantar fasciitis or heel bursitis. However, there may be slight swelling present in a stress fracture, and there is usually pain on the sides of the heels as opposed to the bottom.

Because of the irregular shape of the heel bone, these injuries may be difficult to detect on normal X ray (Figure 4.5), and a bone scan may be required to confirm if a stress fracture is present.

Once a stress fracture is diagnosed, treatment consists of stopping all weight-bearing exercise for at least six weeks. A cast is usually not necessary, but crutches may be required for a few weeks if it is too painful for you to walk or stand. As is the case with most heel injuries, including stress fractures, you can still maintain fitness by cross-training with nonweight-bearing exercises such as bicycling, pool running, and swimming.

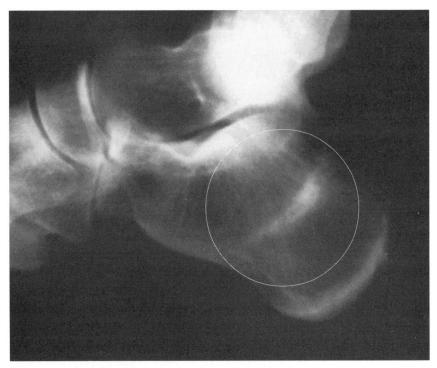

Figure 4.5: X ray showing a stress fracture of the heel

Nerve Entrapments

Although uncommon, irritation to the nerves on the inside of the heel can also result in heel pain. The most common nerves affected are the posterior tibial nerve on the side of the ankle or one of its branches, the medial calcaneal nerve. The tissue surrounding these nerves can become swollen or entrapped due to tendonitis, varicose veins, or overpronation. When the posterior tibial nerve is affected, the condition is known as tarsal tunnel syndrome. Symptoms include numbness, a sensation of pins and needles, or shooting pain into the foot or leg.

The diagnosis of a nerve entrapment may involve a nerve conduction velocity test or magnetic resonance imaging (MRI). Treatment is usually geared towards reducing the inflammation around the nerve and controlling the factors that may have led to the condition. As with other heel problems, surgery should be contemplated only as a last resort.

Medical Heel Pain

Although most heel pain in active individuals is related to overuse, biomechanical abnormalities, or impact-related causes, some heel pain can be due to diseases or problems that originate in other parts of the body. Medical conditions such as gout, diabetes, and certain types of arthritis can affect the heel before showing signs elsewhere in the body. When symptoms are not consistent with biomechanical heel pain, or when discomfort is not relieved by conservative treatment, your sports medicine physician may want to order additional tests to determine whether or not your heel pain could be medically related.

Most heel pain, like other overuse injuries, is the result of excessive activity, improper or worn-out footwear, or biomechanical abnormalities of the lower extremities. If self-care does not provide relief and your pain lasts longer than seven days, gets worse, or recurs, an evaluation by your sports medicine physician will be helpful in determining whether additional forms of treatment are necessary before you can return to full activity. ◢

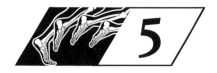

All About Achilles

THE ACHILLES TENDON IS THE STRONGEST TENDON IN THE BODY, yet because of the great amount of stress this tendon is subjected to, it is prone to fitness injuries. These injuries can range from tendonitis to a complete rupture and can significantly limit your participation in sports during the healing process. However, you can often prevent Achilles injuries or lessen their severity with early recognition and treatment.

The Achilles tendon is a thick, cord-like structure that inserts into the back of the heel bone (calcaneus). Tendons attach muscle to bone, and the Achilles tendon joins the two calf muscles, the gastrocnemius and soleus, to the heel (Figure 5.1). Most Achilles injuries occur approximately two inches above the heel bone, an area of the tendon that has a relatively poor blood supply. This poor blood sup-

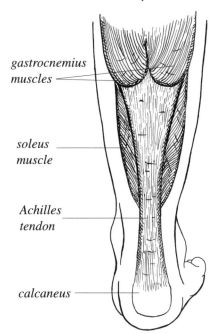

Figure 5.1: The Achilles tendon joins the gastrocnemius and the soleus to the heel

ply also accounts for the relatively long time these injuries often take to heal. The most common injuries to the Achilles area are tendonitis, calf muscle tear (tennis leg), and tendon rupture.

Achilles Tendonitis

Achilles tendonitis is an inflammation of either the sheath surrounding the tendon or the tendon itself. Symptoms usually include a burning pain or tenderness approximately two inches above the heel bone. You may also detect mild to moderate swelling and, in chronic cases, a thickening of the tendon when compared to the opposite leg.

There are many causes of Achilles tendonitis, but the most common are training errors, calf muscle inflexibility, and biomechanical abnormalities. Training errors include increasing your mileage or workout intensity too suddenly or changing your running terrain too abruptly. Inflexibility of the calf muscles can result from improper or inadequate stretching or overstrengthening of the calf muscles. This inflexibility can also be due to wearing high-heeled shoes that tend to shorten the muscle–tendon complex. Biomechanical abnormalities that can lead to Achilles problems include overpronation (flattening of the arch) and leg length differences.

All of the above factors contribute to increased stress on the tendon, resulting in microtears, inflammation, and pain. Because of the poor blood supply to this area, early treatment is necessary to prevent a chronic injury. Initial treatment should include reducing or stopping your sports activities for a period of time. During this time you should be icing the back of your Achilles two to three times a day for 15 minutes. You can use ice packs or massage the area with water frozen in paper cups. Under no circumstance should cortisone be used in the area of the Achilles tendon. Although cortisone will reduce the inflammation, it can slow or prevent the healing of the tendon fibers, possibly resulting in a tendon rupture.

A common mistake in rehabilitating an Achilles tendon injury is to "stretch the Achilles tendon," which usually results in continued irritation of the injured tendon. Instead, you should concentrate your stretching on the gastrocnemius and soleus muscle in a gradual, progressive fashion. Using heel lifts can also help take stress off the tendon; however, be sure to place lifts in both shoes or you may develop an imbalance that leads to other injuries.

Another type of Achilles tendonitis that can occur in active individuals is insertional Achilles tendonitis. This injury is caused by the same mechanisms that lead to classic Achilles tendonitis, but the pain and damage to the tendon occur where the tendon inserts into the heel bone instead of above it. The chronic irritation to the Achilles insertion can sometimes cause the formation of a bone spur (Figure 5.2). If you have this condition, you may notice a thickening in the back of the heel and tenderness directly behind the heel. This condition can also result in an inflammation of a small, fluid-filled sac located in this area called the retrocalcaneal bursa. This bursa normally helps cushion the Achilles from the underlying bone; however, chronic irritation can cause this area to become painful.

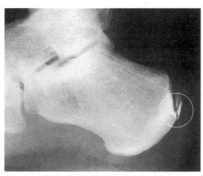

Figure 5.2: Achilles calcification

As mentioned earlier, Achilles tendonitis can be slow to heal. If your pain lingers or gets worse, you should seek a sports medicine physician for a more thorough evaluation. Treatment for this condition can range from temporary heel lifts, calf stretching, and forms of physical therapy, including massage therapy, to cast immobilization for a period of time if you do not respond to other forms of treatment. If biomechanical abnormalities such as overpronation, leg length differences, or other structural problems are suspected, you should undergo a lower extremity biomechanical examination. In these circumstances, orthotics may reduce the stress to the Achilles tendon area and thus relieve your pain.

The treatment for insertional Achilles tendonitis is similar to the treament for Achilles tendonitis. In most circumstances, even if a bone spur or calcification is present, surgery is a last option when all other methods have failed.

Calf Muscle Tear (Tennis Leg)

Achilles tendonitis is often caused by overuse, whereas calf muscle tears and tendon ruptures are usually the result of a traumatic injury. A calf muscle tear is actually a misnomer; the injury usually occurs where the calf muscles join the Achilles tendon on the inside part of the leg about two thirds of the way down from the knee.

This injury often happens when you push off on the leg while reaching for a tennis shot — hence the name "tennis leg." Symptoms of a calf muscle tear include the sensation of being hit in the back of the leg, followed by pain and swelling in the affected area. The swelling may even extend into the ankle area. Standing and walking are usually painful.

Initial treatment for a calf muscle tear should consist of RICE: rest, ice, compression, and elevation. Your sports medicine physician needs to evaluate your injury to make sure the tendon itself has not been torn. In most cases reduced activity, physical therapy and massage therapy, and gradual stretching can speed the healing process.

Achilles Tendon Rupture

Rupture of the Achilles tendon, although not that common, is a very serious injury. It usually occurs from a sudden, explosive movement such as reaching for a tennis shot, chasing a basketball rebound, or sprinting. Usually a person suffering this injury will describe the feeling of having been hit in the back of the leg and hearing a pop or snap. The pain is usually severe, walking is difficult, and it is impossible to stand on the toes of the affected leg.

Achilles tendon ruptures are most common in individuals aged 35 to 55. Very often the injured person has a history of tight calf muscles or previous Achilles tendonitis; the lack of a proper warm-up is also common prior to this injury. The rupture most frequently occurs in the same location as Achilles tendonitis, two inches above the heel bone, and may be partial or complete.

Immediate evaluation by a sports medicine physician is necessary to prevent further damage and possible permanent injury. Partial ruptures can usually be treated successfully with a cast; however, complete ruptures may require surgery.

Preventing Achilles Tendon Injuries

Achilles tendon injuries can be very serious and heal slowly. However, warming up sufficiently, maintaining adequate lower extremity flexibility, and training sensibly can prevent many of these injuries. Warming up is important for any exercise, as this prepares the body for the activity it is about to undergo. Insufficient warm-up may subject tendons and muscles to excessive stretch and result in injury.

Achilles injuries can have a significant impact on your training programs. Sensible training can prevent Achilles injuries by allowing the body to adapt to the increasing demands placed on the tendon. This can be accomplished by gradually increasing your walking and running distance and training intensity. The most important measure for avoiding Achilles tendon injuries is maintaining adequate lower extremity flexibility. Normal activities such as standing, sitting, and wearing shoes with a heel height greater than one inch contribute to tightness of the muscles and tendon in the back of the leg. A regular stretching program that emphasizes the gastrocnemius and soleus muscles of the calf can play a great role in preventing downtime from an Achilles tendon injury. When symptoms of an Achilles problem do occur, prompt recognition and early treatment can reduce the time it takes for these injuries to heal. ▰

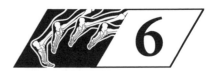

If It's Not Shin Splints, What Is It?

THE SHIN AREA IS SUBJECT TO A GREAT DEAL OF STRESS DURING sports and fitness activities and, thus, is prone to many overuse injuries. The term "shin splints" is often used to describe the soreness that can affect this area. However, the term is not a specific diagnosis but rather a general name for a variety of conditions with different causes.

The shin refers to the front area of the leg between the ankle and the knee (Figure 6.1) and includes the tibia and fibula (leg bones); the muscles of the leg, which are divided into compartments; and nerves and blood vessels. Shin pain can result from injury to any of these structures, either by direct trauma or overuse. Overuse injuries in this area can be caused by overtraining, hard exercise surfaces, muscle imbalance or inflexibility, and abnormal biomechanical function of the lower extremities. For any of these shin problems to be treated successfully, you need to have an accurate diagnosis based on the history of the injury, an examination of the area, and special tests if needed.

Muscle and Tendon Injuries

The muscles and tendons that make up the shin area include the anterior tibial muscle and tendon on the front part of the leg, the posterior tibial muscles and tendon on the inside (medial aspect) of the leg and the peroneus longus and peroneus brevis muscles and tendons on the outside (lateral aspect) of the leg. These muscles and tendons work together to control motion of the lower extremity during activity.

PERRY H. JULIEN, DPM

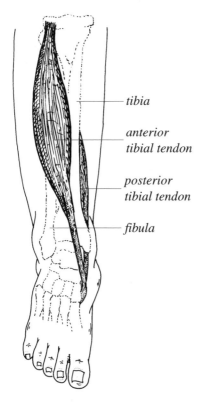

tibia

anterior
tibial tendon

posterior
tibial tendon

fibula

Figure 6.1: Shin anatomy

The anterior tibial muscle and tendon help bring the foot upward to clear the ground when you run and walk. The posterior tibial muscle and tendon resist the flattening of the arch and reduce the rate of pronation as the foot strikes the ground. The muscles on the outside of the leg (peroneus longus and peroneus brevis) oppose the posterior tibial muscle and tendon and help prevent the foot from rolling out excessively.

Injuries affecting one of these muscle–tendon combinations will usually result in tenderness over a two- to six-inch area overlying the tendon. The discomfort is usually worse at the onset of activity and will sometimes diminish as the muscle and tendon warm up and stretch. After activity, as the muscles and tendons cool down and tighten up, the pain will often return. There is usually no pain at rest.

Anterior tibial tendon shin pain is often due to tight calf muscles. Tight calf muscles add stress on the anterior tibial tendon to help flex the foot and ankle up during activity. The posterior tibial tendon is often aggravated by overpronation or excessive breakdown of your shoes, resulting in increased stress on the inside of the leg. Shin pain as a result of peroneal tendon injuries can be related to excessive wear on the outside of an athletic shoe or may be due to alterations in lower extremity biomechanical function.

Early treatment for shin pain due to muscle or tendon problems involves the RICE principle of rest, ice, compression, and elevation. In most overuse injuries, the rest and ice are the most important components, as muscle and tendon injuries that affect the shin do not tend to swell. Rest reduces the amount of stress to the area and allows the injury to heal. In many cases, cutting back on the length or intensity of your training, changing the surfaces on which you exercise, and replacing shoes that are worn-out will aid the recovery process. Apply ice for 15 minutes every few hours to help reduce inflammation in the area.

An important consideration in both the rehabilitation and prevention of an anterior tibial tendon shin injury involves maintaining the correct balance between the muscles in the lower leg. Tightness in the calf muscles will often predispose you to injuries either directly or indirectly. A daily stretching routine that emphasizes the calf muscles is one of the best forms of preventive medicine and should decrease the likelihood that you will suffer from this or other common overuse injuries.

In situations where pain persists, your sports medicine physician may recommend other treatments, including physical therapy; massage therapy; and orthotics, if the tendon injury is thought to be a result of biomechanical factors affecting the lower leg.

Periostitis

The periosteum is a thin membrane that surrounds bones and plays a role in bone nutrition and repair. The periosteum of the tibia and fibula is also the insertion point for some of the muscles of the lower leg. When overstressed, the muscular insertions may irritate or tear off the periosteum, resulting in inflammation called periostitis.

Periostitis of the shin area is most painful when you exercise, but a dull ache may remain even after a period of rest. The pain is usually located deep in the shin area and along the shaft of the bones. In most instances, the pain covers an area of approximately two to six inches, similar to that seen in tendonitis.

The causes of this injury are similar to the causes of muscle and tendon strains; in fact, left untreated, a muscle strain may progress to periostitis. The diagnosis is usually based on the history of the injury and a physical examination. In some cases, there may also be subtle changes in X rays of the area where the muscle attaches to the bone.

The treatment for periostitis is similar to that used for muscle strains; activities that affect the legs, such as running, may need to be restricted. A biomechanical exam of your foot and leg function may reveal abnormalities that can predispose you to developing this injury, but you can take steps to correct these abnormalities, speed recovery, and prevent recurrence of the injury.

Stress Fractures

Stress fractures of the tibia and fibula are another cause of shin pain in active individuals. In contrast to muscle–tendon injury and periostitis, someone with a stress fracture can usually point to a very specific area on the bone that is tender. The pain from this injury is almost always present during strenuous activity but may also be noticeable when you walk or stand.

Stress fractures result from low-level repetitive trauma to a specific area of the bone. In the leg bones, these injuries usually occur one-third or two-thirds of the way from the knee to the ankle.

Our bones adapt to the increased demands of exercise by laying down more bone and getting stronger. However, if not given time to accommodate the additional stress, the bone will develop small cracks, resulting in a fracture.

Most often, the bone does not move out of place when a stress fracture occurs, which initially makes the injury difficult to diagnosis by X ray. As the bone begins to heal, new bone called callus begins to appear. This new bone can be seen on X ray four to six weeks after the injury occurs. In many instances, however, the tibia and fibula may not show callus formation, even though the bone is healing. A more reliable way to confirm a stress fracture is a bone scan, a test that involves injecting a small amount of a radioactive dye into the body, which then makes its way to areas of bone injury. The leg is then scanned two hours later, and a stress fracture shows up as a black dot (Figure 6.2). This test can reveal a stress fracture two days after it occurs, even when X rays appear normal.

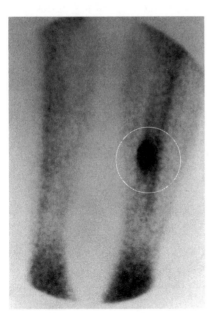

Figure 6.2: Bone scan indicating a stress fracture of the tibia

Once diagnosed, treatment for a stress fracture involves discontinuing any weight-bearing fitness activities for six weeks to six months. The average healing time is about eight weeks. In many cases, a cast or crutches will not be necessary; however, a removable brace may provide support. Cross-training such as swimming and pool running can help you maintain fitness during the recovery period.

In some cases, stress fractures may be the result of a structural or biomechanical abnormality that places too much pressure on a specific area of the leg. In these instances, orthotics may help prevent a recurrence of a stress fracture.

Compartment Syndrome

The muscles of the lower leg are grouped in four sections called compartments, which are formed by fibrous tissue called fascia. In addition to muscles, each compartment contains nerves and blood vessels. During physical activity, muscles usually expand, and these compartments also expand slightly. However, if the muscles expand beyond the point that the compartments can accommodate, excessive pressure on the muscles and structures in the compartment can result in significant pain.

Compartment syndrome may be due to a congenitally tight compartment, from overuse of the muscle, or overdevelopment of the muscles in the compartment.

The pain resulting from exercise-induced compartment syndrome is usually described as a deep ache in the muscle area rather than near the bone. The pain appears shortly after exercise begins and generally improves rapidly once the activity has ceased. The pain, however, is usually significant enough that you have to stop whatever activity you are doing. Over time, symptoms may progress to numbness and muscle weakness in the leg and foot caused by pressure being placed on the nerves in the compartment.

When compartment syndrome is suspected, your sports medicine physician may recommend a test that measures the pressure in the affected compartment before and after exercise. An elevation of this pressure usually confirms the diagnosis.

Conservative treatment for compartment syndrome may involve minimizing stress to the involved leg. This could involve a change in activity or training surface, rest, stretching, anti-inflammatory medication, and the use of orthotics to control any biomechanical abnormalities. These steps may relieve the symptoms and allow the muscles in the compartment to return to normal. To prevent a recurrence, you may have to alter your training and manage other factors that contributed to your injury.

When conservative treatment is ineffective, you may require surgery, which involves making a small incision in the fascia of the affected compartment(s) to allow the muscles more room to expand.

Although uncommon, compartment syndrome is another cause of chronic shin and leg pain that, once diagnosed, can be treated, allowing you to return to pain-free activity.

Many of the shin injuries described in this chapter are the result of the body not having enough time to adapt to increased demands placed upon it. By establishing a reasonable training program that involves a gradual increase in exercise intensity, proper stretching and strengthening, and attention to proper shoe gear and technique, you can prevent many of these overuse injuries. Have your sports medicine physician evaluate any pain that persists longer than seven days with self-treatment, gets worse, or recurs. ◢◤

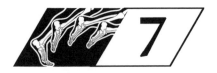

Tendon Injuries of the Foot and Leg

TENDONS ARE FIBROUS, CORD-LIKE STRUCTURES THAT ATTACH muscles to bones. Their names are usually derived from the muscles they attach. Most tendons are covered by sheaths that help them glide and provide them with nutrition.

Tendon injuries can range from mild strains to complete tears. When a tendon is strained or becomes inflamed, the condition is called tendonitis. Excessive, repetitive movements or sudden forces that irritate the tendon or its sheath are common causes of tendonitis.

When stretched too far, a tendon can tear or rupture. Symptoms of a tendon rupture include severe pain, swelling, bruising, and the inability to move the area of the body that the affected muscles or tendons control.

There are many tendons in the body, but some are more prone to injury because of the greater force to which they are subjected. In the lower extremity, the posterior tibial, anterior tibial, peroneal, and Achilles tendons are the most frequently injured because of the role they play in supporting and controlling the foot and leg during sports and fitness activities.

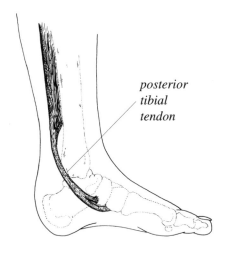

posterior tibial tendon

Figure 7.1: Posterior tibial tendon

Posterior Tibial Tendon

The posterior tibial tendon, located on the inside of the ankle, runs behind the ankle bone (malleolus) (Figure 7.1). Its main function is to resist overpronation (flattening of the arch) that can occur when you walk or run. A flat arch or over-pronated foot can lead to posterior tibial tendonitis because of the increased stress placed on this tendon in an effort to support the arch. Dysfunction or rupture of the posterior tibial tendon can also lead to a progressive flattening of the arch over time.

Anterior Tibial Tendon

The anterior tibial muscle and tendon, located in front of the leg (Figure 7.2), help lift the foot when you walk or run and also slow the front part of the foot (forefoot) to keep it from hitting the ground too rapidly. Both running and walking strengthen the calf muscles more than those of the shin. The resulting imbalance can lead to anterior tibial tendonitis as the muscles and tendons on the front of the shin have to work harder to lift the foot, especially if the calf muscles are tight. This is common when running or walking up and down hills.

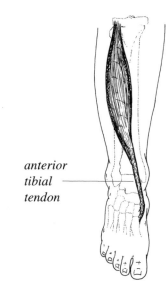

anterior tibial tendon

Figure 7.2: Anterior tibial tendon

Peroneal Tendons

The peroneal muscles and tendons, located on the outside of the leg and foot, consist of the peroneus longus and the peroneus brevis (Figure 7.3). These tendons support the outside of the ankle and stabilize the foot during activity. They are most often injured by twisting or turning the ankle outward, running on irregular surfaces, or wearing shoes with excessive wear on the outside (lateral) portion of the heel. When an athletic shoe wears down, the foot has a tendency to strike more to the outside, placing in-

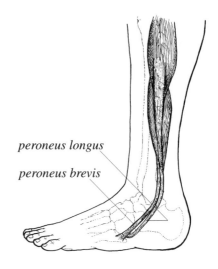

Figure 7.3: Peroneal tendons

creased stress on the peroneal muscles and tendons as they try to prevent the ankle from rolling out too much.

Achilles Tendon

The Achilles tendon (Figure 7.4) joins the two calf muscles (gastrocnemius and soleus) to the back of the heel bone (calcaneus). One of the strongest tendons in the body, it is still prone to injury because of the tremendous stress placed upon it with every step.

Achilles tendonitis usually occurs because of overtraining or calf muscle inflexibility. It can also result from abnormal lower extremity biomechanics such as overpronation, which places excessive force on the tendon.

The Achilles tendon is most commonly injured approximately two inches above the heel bone. Because this area is also the loca-

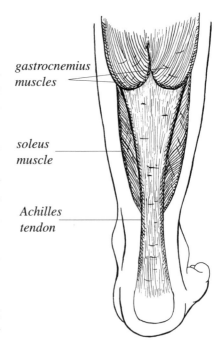

Figure 7.4: Achilles tendon

tion of the tendon's poorest blood supply, Achilles tendon injuries can heal very slowly.

Achilles tendon tears can be very serious and usually occur as a result of a sudden movement such as reaching for a tennis shot or sprinting without proper warm-up. An Achilles tendon tear requires immediate attention to avoid damaging consequences.

Symptoms of Tendon Injuries

Tendonitis can occur gradually from repetitive microtrauma or can result from a sudden movement. Initial symptoms can include pain with activity, mild swelling, and occasionally a crackling sensation over the tendon as it moves. This last symptom is caused by a collection of fluid between the tendon and tendon sheath.

In general, the symptoms of tendonitis may improve during the course of activity. This is due in part to the warming up and gradual stretching of the tendon, which takes stress off the injured area; however, the tendon will usually tighten up and cause a significant increase in discomfort after you are done with the activity. If this injury cycle is allowed to persist without treatment, the tendon or sheath may thicken, resulting in chronic discomfort and a decrease in flexibility. If left untreated, chronic tendonitis can predispose you to further injury or possible tendon rupture.

Diagnosis and Treatment

The early treatment of any sports injury, including tendonitis, should follow the RICE principle of rest, ice, compression, and elevation. The amount of rest required for tendonitis depends on the severity of the injury. Often "rest" can incorporate some form of cross-training so you can maintain your aerobic fitness and strength. Apply ice for 15 minutes several times a day. Compression and elevation are often not necessary in tendonitis, as these injuries do not usually swell. However, if swelling is present, elevate your leg above the level of your heart and use an elastic wrap to reduce swelling.

In mild cases of tendonitis, several days of RICE therapy should reduce symptoms and allow you to return to activity. In more severe cases, the use of oral nonsteroidal anti-inflammatories, physical therapy or massage therapy, and temporary immobilization may speed recovery.

When the pain does not go away in seven days, worsens, or recurs, seek evaluation from a sports medicine physician. Injuries such as stress fractures, ligament tears, and joint injuries can sometimes mimic tendonitis and may require more aggressive care. Severe pain and swelling can also indicate a tendon tear or rupture, which may need immediate attention to prevent further damage to the area.

If more aggressive medical attention is needed, your physician may recommend temporary bracing or immobilization to treat a severe tendonitis. If a tendon tear is suspected, your physician may recommend a diagnostic test such as magnetic resonance imaging (MRI). An MRI allows the muscles, tendons, and ligaments to be visualized, unlike X rays, which show only bone injuries. This added information will help your sports medicine physician make a more precise diagnosis and subsequent treatment plan for a tendon injury.

Following correct training and exercise protocols can often prevent tendonitis as well as other sports-related overuse injuries. You should always warm up slowly before beginning any fitness activity and follow a regular routine of stretching and flexibility exercises. A gradual increase in exercise intensity allows the body to adapt to the increased demands being placed upon it, resulting in fewer injuries. Selecting the right footwear can also minimize stress to specific muscles and tendons.

Imbalances such as overpronation, leg length differences, and hereditary bone structure problems may need to be addressed with some form of biomechanical control such as orthotics. These orthotics place the foot and leg in a more biomechanically correct position to allow the bones, muscles, and tendons to function more efficiently and to lessen the stress on specific areas of the lower extremity. Orthotics can help treat tendonitis as well as prevent other problems from developing in susceptible individuals.

The benefits of regular exercise far outweigh the occasional risk of injury. By training wisely, you can avoid many of these problems. However, when an injury does occur, early evaluation and treatment can, in most cases, get you going again quickly. ◢

8

Metatarsal Maladies

ACTIVE INDIVIDUALS FREQUENTLY COMPLAIN ABOUT PAIN IN THE ball of the foot or around the toes. Physicians often call this condition metatarsalgia, which is a general term for discomfort in this area. However, it is important to determine the precise cause of your symptoms because the more specific the diagnosis is, the more focused the treatment for the problem can be.

The ball of the foot is made up of the five metatarsal bones that form part of both the longitudinal and transverse arches (Figure 8.1). Several ligaments, muscles, and tendons surround this area and help the foot perform its role in weight-bearing and propulsion. Small blood vessels and nerves also run parallel to the metatarsal bones and extend into the toes.

Injuries to the metatarsal region may be the result of direct trauma, overuse, abnormal lower extremity biomechanics, or inappropriate footwear. Among the more common injuries are metatarsal bursitis, Morton's neuroma, stress fractures, and sesamoiditis. Early recognition and treatment of any of these problems can shorten your recovery.

Metatarsal Bursitis

Metatarsal bursitis is an inflammation of the fluid-filled sacs known as bursas, located underneath the metatarsal bones. These bursas act as a cushion for the ball of the foot and can be injured when excessive pressure such as the repetitive pounding of fitness activities is placed on them. Those who participate in sports that require landing on the midfoot or toes are more prone to this injury.

Other contributing factors include worn-out footwear cushioning, an inadequate fat pad on the ball of the foot, a plantarflexed (lowered) metatarsal bone, and Morton's foot. Morton's foot is a genetic condition in which the second metatarsal is abnormally long and thus causes greater stress to be placed on this area. Symptoms of metatarsal bursitis include tenderness on the ball of the foot, directly under one or more of the metatarsal bones. This injury most commonly affects the second, third, or fourth metatarsal bone. There may also be some mild swelling and skin callus formation. The pain is usually most noticeable just before you push off your toes.

Initial treatment for metatarsal bursitis should include icing the area two or three times a day for 15 minutes to reduce inflammation and adding some form of shock-absorbing shoe insert to decrease pressure to the area. If this treatment is unsuccessful, various types of padding can be used to disperse weight from the injured metatarsal while it is healing. A metatarsal pad made of felt, foam, or other material can be placed behind the pain-

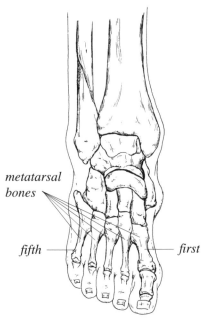

Figure 8.1: Metatarsal anatomy

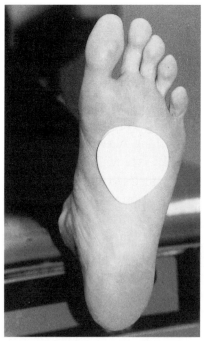

Figure 8.2: Metatarsal pad placement

ful area, either in the shoe or directly on the foot (Figure 8.2), to reduce pressure in the painful area. You should wear this type of padding throughout the day, not just when you exercise.

In cases where the problem is due, in part, to abnormal biomechanics, you can use orthotics to alter the pressure distribution on the bottom of the foot. If necessary, your sports medicine physician can incorporate a metatarsal pad into your orthotic as well to relieve pain and prevent a recurrence of this injury.

Morton's Neuroma

A neuroma is the thickening of a nerve that occurs as a result of chronic irritation or trauma. Although a neuroma can theoretically occur anywhere on the foot, the most common location in active individuals is between the third and fourth metatarsals (Figure 8.3). A neuroma in this area is called Morton's neuroma, named after Dr. T. G. Morton, who first described this problem. This injury is not to be confused with Morton's foot, which is a long second metatarsal and was identified by and named after Dr. Dudley Morton.

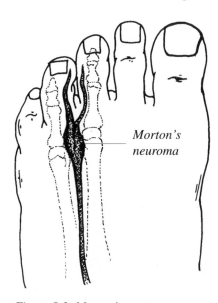

Morton's neuroma

Morton's neuroma results from pressure on the nerve, often created by a compression of the third and fourth metatarsal bones. This compression can be due to a narrow toe box in a shoe or thick socks that create a tight fit in the forefoot. Our feet swell slightly during activity, which may result in a seemingly well-fitting shoe becoming too snug during prolonged fitness activity. Other possible causes include direct injury to the metatarsal area and biomechanical factors such as overpronation.

Figure 8.3: Morton's neuroma, most commonly occurring between the third and fourth metatarsals

A neuroma often feels like a sharp or burning pain in the ball of the foot with pain or a pins and needles sensation that radiates to the third and fourth toes. These symptoms can also be present between the second and third toes. You may also feel a clicking sensation in this area during activity and a feeling that your socks are bunching up in the shoe. Removing your shoes and massaging the metatarsal region may relieve the symptoms. However, they usually recur shortly after resuming activity.

Self-treatment for a neuroma involves first making sure that all of your footwear — not just your athletic shoes — fits correctly. You can also place a cotton ball between the affected toes to take pressure off the nerve by separating the metatarsal bones. If pain persists despite this self-treatment, injection therapy can often alleviate the pain. In a small number of cases, when these conservative approaches do not relieve the pain, your sports medicine physician may recommend surgery to remove the enlarged nerve.

Metatarsal Stress Fractures

Stress fractures are the result of cumulative microtrauma placed on an area of bone over time, which causes the bone to fatigue and fracture. Overtraining is often the cause of stress fractures, because individuals do not give the bone enough time to repair after stress. Biomechanical abnormalities such as overpronation can also contribute to stress fractures.

The metatarsal bones are especially prone to stress fractures because of the forces placed on them during running. The second, third, and fourth metatarsals are most often affected because of their anatomic relationship with other bones in the foot. Stress fractures of the fifth metatarsal are less common and can take significantly longer to heal.

Early symptoms of a stress fracture include pain during activity, mild to moderate swelling, and pain over a small area of the bone. Standard X rays may be normal in the early stages of this injury. Over time, bone callus may form (Figure 8.4), indicating the start of the

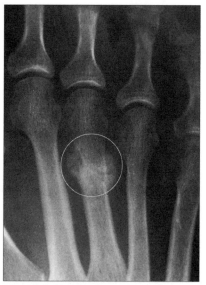

Figure 8.4: A healing metatarsal stress fracture showing bone callus

healing process and confirming the presence of a stress fracture. In some circumstances a diagnostic test called a bone scan may be necessary to provide a definitive diagnosis.

The treatment for a stress fracture involves discontinuing all weight-bearing fitness activities until the fracture heals, which could take between six weeks and six months. Most stress fractures, however, will heal in about eight weeks, and often a cast is not necessary. You can cross-train with activities such as pool running, swimming, and cycling to maintain aerobic fitness.

Sesamoid Injuries

Pain occurring on the ball of the foot just behind the big toe often involves two small sesamoid bones that lie underneath the first metatarsal. These bones are imbedded in tendons and act as a pulley system to flex the big toe (hallux). Sesamoid bones can be bruised (sesamoiditis) or fractured (Figure 8.5) when excessive pressure is placed on the ball of the foot. The symptoms of sesamoiditis usually include pain on the bottom of the foot just behind the big toe joint that is present when you apply pressure to the area or when you flex the toe upwards. The area may also be swollen and warm.

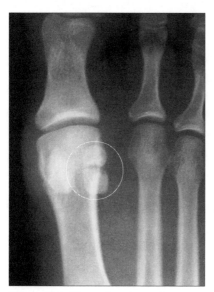

Figure 8.5: X ray showing a fracture of one of the sesamoid bones

Icing this location and using accommodative padding can often take pressure off this area to allow healing to take place. As long as the area underneath the sesamoids is protected and you don't experience any symptoms, you can often continue with fitness activities. If the pain persists, a soft cast or injection therapy may be recommended. You can also use orthotics that incorporate modifications to keep pressure off this area and reduce the risk of a recurrence.

Sesamoid bones are also prone to stress fractures, because they are subjected to repetitive low-level stress. Since the sesamoid bones are prominent on the bottom of the feet, they are often exposed to this type of overuse trauma.

In cases of sesamoid stress fractures, X rays will typically show the sesamoid bone in two or three pieces. However, this diagnosis can be complicated by the fact that the sesamoid bones sometimes occur in two or more pieces, a normal condition called bipartite or multipartite sesamoids. This situation is a result of irregular bone formation in childhood. When the existence of a stress fracture is in question, a bone scan will usually give an accurate diagnosis.

Whereas sesamoiditis may respond to treatment in two or four weeks, sesamoid stress fractures can sometimes take a few months to heal. The sesamoid bones do not have a very good blood supply and therefore heal slowly when fractured. In many instances the bones will not join together but will heal with a fibrous type of tissue between the fragments.

As long as the area underneath the sesamoid bones is protected, athletes with sesamoiditis or a sesamoid stress fracture can usually continue with their fitness pursuits. They may need to replace activities that result in significant pressure on the ball of the foot with a form of lower-impact exercise. If removing pressure from the area does not relieve the pain, and if conservative care does not provide relief, the affected sesamoid bone may need to be removed surgically. Removing a sesamoid bone can affect the position of the toe, so surgery should be used only as a last resort.

You can avoid sesamoid injuries by wearing shoes with adequate cushioning under the ball of your foot and replacing shoes when they are worn-out. Also, try to avoid hard, unforgiving training surfaces to reduce stress in this area.

In situations where the sesamoid area is chronically injured and painful, a podiatrist may recommend orthotics to redistribute the pressure placed on the sesamoids.

There are other conditions such as arthritis, tendon injuries, and assorted bone problems that can cause metatarsal pain. If you experience a persistent pain in this area, an evaluation by your sports medicine physician may be in order. ◢

9

The Big Toe Joint

EACH FOOT CONSISTS OF 28 BONES AND 55 JOINTS THAT WORK together to support and propel us in all our activities. The first metatarsal phalangeal joint (first MPJ), formed by the first metatarsal bone and the hallux (big toe), plays a key role as you push off the front part of your foot and move forward. The first MPJ requires about 60 degrees of upward bend (dorsiflexion) to function properly during toe-off. This motion requires the integrated work of the metatarsal, hallux, and sesamoid bones; the joint capsule; ligaments; and six tendons.

During fitness activities, our feet often encounter forces between one-and-a-half to three times our body weight, and problems affecting the motion or position of this joint can result in pain in the joint itself or elsewhere as the body tries to compensate. The two most common first MPJ problems are hallux valgus (bunion) and hallux limitus.

Hallux Valgus

A bunion appears as an enlargement or bump on the outside of the first MPJ (Figure 9.1). In actuality, this bony protrusion indicates that a misalignment or partial dislocation of the joint has taken place (Figure 9.2).

Most bunion deformities result from muscle and tendon imbalances around the first MPJ. These imbalances may be due to abnormal biomechanics such as overpronation or from an individual's specific foot structure. The effect of the imbalances, however, is a progressive

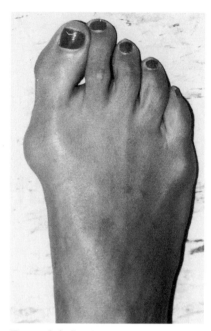

Figure 9.1: Bunion

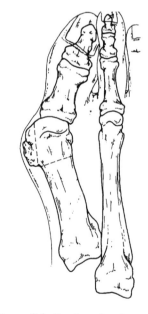

Figure 9.2: Bunion showing misalignment of bones

alteration of the joint position. Tight or poorly fitting shoes by themselves do not usually cause a bunion to form; however, if your shoes press against the prominent bone, you may feel discomfort and the deformity may increase in size over time.

The size of the bunion deformity does not always correlate to the level of pain you experience. Bunions do not always cause pain, so choosing shoes with a wide toe box to avoid irritation can prevent bunion problems in the future. If a bunion does start to become painful, switching to shoes with a wider toe box may take enough pressure off the inflamed area to relieve the discomfort. Using bunion shields, available in pharmacies, can also reduce pressure irritation.

As the bunion enlarges, you may also develop pain under the second metatarsal on the ball of the foot. A bunion elevates the first metatarsal bone slightly, which can increase the pressure underneath the adjacent bones. In these circumstances, an orthotic can often redistribute the pressure under the lesser metatarsals and relieve the discomfort.

When a bunion deformity becomes painful enough to limit your activity and lifestyle, and attempts at shoe modification and accommodative padding have not relieved the discomfort, surgery to correct

PERRY H. JULIEN, DPM

the bunion deformity may be indicated. Bunion surgery may also be recommended when there is an obvious progression of the bunion deformity over time. In most circumstances, bunion pain is a result of the pressure or irritation from the prominence at the first MPJ. The pain can also come from arthritis that can develop in the joint as the toe drifts over. In this case, the misalignment of the joint can cause damage to the cartilage surfaces that form the first MPJ, making it painful to move the toe up and down and aggravating the joint while you walk or exercise.

The goal of most bunion surgeries is not to remove the prominent bone but rather to realign the joint. If the joint surfaces are realigned, the bony protrusion or bump should disappear. Depending on your age, activity level, and severity of the bunion deformity, there are many different surgical procedures that can be used to correct bunions. Most of these procedures involve making a surgical break in the bone or taking out a small wedge of bone to achieve good joint realignment.

Following any type of surgical procedure, the primary concern of active individuals is the amount of time required for recovery. With bunion surgery this varies from person to person, but in general a cast is not necessary after surgery, and you can start some form of cross-training that does not place excessive stress on the feet 2 to 3 weeks after surgery. Before you can return to full weight-bearing exercise, complete bone healing must take place, which could take 8 to 12 weeks.

Following bunion surgery, your doctor may recommend that you use orthotics in your shoes to prevent a recurrence of the bunion by controlling any abnormal biomechanical motion that may have contributed to the problem in the first place.

Hallux Limitus

Another problem that can affect the first MPJ is hallux limitus, a limitation of upward motion (dorsiflexion) of the big toe that can occur as a result of injury to the joint or inherited foot structure. The first MPJ requires between 55 and 65 degrees of dorsiflexion to allow for normal foot motion during activity. A long first metatarsal, an elevated first metatarsal, or excessive motion of the bones on the medial aspect (inside) of the foot can reduce the range of motion at the first MPJ. Over time, the resulting microtrauma can cause small bone spurs to

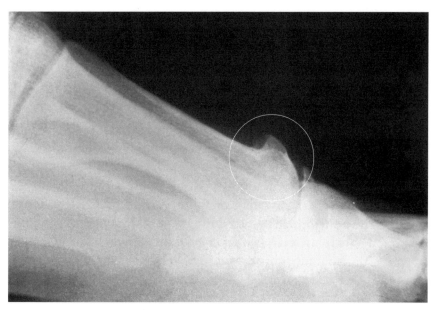

Figure 9.3: Bone spur at the top of the first metatarsal caused by and/or contributing to hallux limitus

develop at the top of the first metatarsal that will further limit motion of the joint (Figure 9.3).

Hallux limitus can also develop from an injury to the bone or cartilage in the joint area, if, for example, an object falls directly on the joint or if the joint surfaces are compressed as a result of kicking something or someone.

Functional hallux limitus is a limitation of joint motion that usually occurs only during weight-bearing activities. In this situation, biomechanical abnormalities such as overpronation can reduce the motion in your first MPJ when you walk or run, which causes the lower extremity to compensate for this lack of motion. Functional hallux limitus is not always associated with the formation of bone spurs, and the joint motion may appear normal when no weight is on the foot.

The early symptoms of hallux limitus may include pain in the joint or the development of bone spurs on the top of the joint, which may be accompanied by swelling or skin irritation from the top of your shoes. If left untreated, the bone spur may enlarge, and small pieces may break off into the joint, which can wear away the smooth cartilage surfaces that normally provide pain-free joint motion.

Even before pain begins to occur at the first MPJ, you may develop symptoms elsewhere as the body attempts to compensate for this lack of motion. The ability to push off your toes may be restricted, which places more pressure on the outside (lateral) part of your foot and causes pain in this region. The alteration in your normal gait cycle can also lead to knee pain, shin pain, Achilles pain, heel pain, and other overuse injuries.

The treatment for hallux limitus runs from range of motion exercises and attempts to increase joint motion to surgery to remove the bone spurs or bone fragments or to repair any structural deformity of the first metatarsal. In cases where significant bony changes have not taken place and your doctor can identify biomechanical irregularities, orthotics with specific modifications can place your foot in a more biomechanically correct position, relieving the stress placed on the first MPJ. This type of early intervention for hallux limitus can prevent the progression of the deformity and avoid further damage to the joint and cartilage.

Joint Arthritis

Joint arthritis occurs when some damage to the joint or its surrounding structures has taken place. First MPJ arthritis can result from direct trauma, overuse stress such as hallux limitus, structural deformities such as bunions, or medical conditions affecting the joints. The most common of these medical conditions is gout.

Gout is a metabolic disease that is caused by an accumulation of uric acid crystals in the joint. The first MPJ is the most common area for a gout attack to occur because of a relative lack of circulation and temperature given its distance from the main circulation of the heart. Symptoms of gout usually occur initially at night and are often accompanied by severe pain, swelling, warmth, and redness around the big toe joint. The accumulation of uric acid crystals causing these symptoms usually results from an overproduction or underexcretion of uric acid in the body.

Attacks of gout often occur after a meal of rich, fatty food and alcohol. Minor traumas such as those associated with overuse syndromes may also precipitate an attack. Dehydration can also play a role, as it tends to concentrate the uric acid crystals in the body.

Treatment of acute gout includes using oral nonsteroidal anti-inflammatories and warm soaks for the affected area. Although the initial inclination is to apply ice to a swollen area, in the case of an acute gout attack, ice can actually cause more uric acid crystals to accumulate in the joint, while heat can sometimes dissolve these crystals and bring them back into circulation.

The symptoms of acute gout can also resemble those associated with trauma or infection. Prompt evaluation by your physician will help determine a precise diagnosis. Although many individuals may suffer one isolated case of gouty arthritis and not have any further recurrences, your doctor's evaluation may help identify factors causing high blood uric acid levels that could contribute to additional episodes. In these circumstances, careful attention to hydration, diet, and the possible use of medications to reduce uric acid levels will help prevent problems in the future.

First metatarsal phalangeal joint injuries are not uncommon in active individuals. When they are caused by biomechanical or structural problems in the foot, appropriate biomechanical control and shoe selection can play a significant role in preventing symptoms from progressing. In situations where, despite your best attempts at controlling these problems, they begin to alter your activities, a sports medicine physician can help you determine the best treatment plan for these foot complaints. ◢

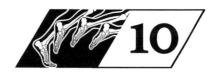

Stress Fractures
Overuse Injuries Affecting Bones

LOWER EXTREMITY SPORTS AND FITNESS INJURIES CAN RANGE FROM overuse syndromes such as tendonitis or plantar fasciitis to traumatic injuries such as ankle sprains and fractures. One of the more frustrating injuries that an active person can suffer is a stress fracture.

Stress fractures are usually seen in individuals who participate in such sports as running, tennis, basketball, and soccer, which subject the foot and leg to repetitive movement. Although a stress fracture represents a true break in a bone, it is considered an overuse injury because it does not result from a single injury but rather from repetitive, low-level stress occurring in a specific area of the bone over time.

Our bones adapt to increased stress by adding more bone cells and getting stronger. A stress fracture occurs when the forces applied to the bone over a period of time exceed the ability of that bone to repair itself. This results in small cracks forming in the bone that may eventually develop into a complete fracture.

The Causes of Stress Fractures

The two most frequent causes of stress fractures in a lower extremity are overtraining and structural or biomechanical imbalances of the foot and leg. Overtraining is usually due to increasing too rapidly the intensity or duration of your sport, which does not allow your bones to adapt to the increased demands being placed on them. A change in the surfaces you exercise on can have the same effect.

A less recognized cause of a stress fracture is a structural or biomechanical abnormality of the lower extremity such as overpronation, leg length differences, ligament laxity (hypermobility), and inflexibility. Any of these conditions can increase the stress being placed on specific areas of the lower extremity and result in a stress fracture. If you are prone to stress fractures and you haven't had any significant alteration in your training, the cause may be a biomechanical or structural abnormality. The "female triad" — amenorrhea or an irregular menstrual cycle, eating disorders, and osteoporosis — can place a woman at a greater risk for stress fractures as well.

Symptoms of a stress fracture include a sharp pain during weight-bearing activities that involve the lower extremity. The pain can often be localized over a very small area of the bone. Depending on the location of the stress fracture, you may also experience swelling or bruising. The pain will also increase as you continue to exercise.

A stress fracture may develop slowly as you try to run through pain, or it may occur suddenly during the course of activity. The bones most often affected by a stress fracture include the tibia and fibula (leg bones), the second, third, and fourth metatarsals, and the calcaneus (heel bone) (Figure 10.1). Less common locations include the navicular bone on the inside of the foot and the fifth metatarsal bone. Stress fractures in these latter two locations tend to take significantly longer to heal because of the limited blood supply to these bones and the presence of tendonous attachments that can add stress on these areas while the fracture is healing.

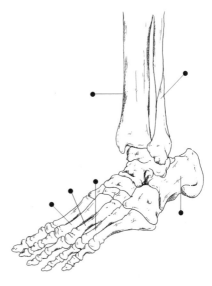

Figure 10.1: Most common locations of stress fractures

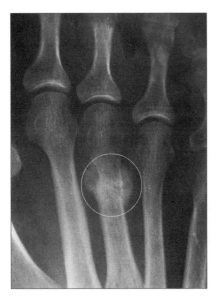

Figure 10.2: Bone callus in a healing metatarsal stress fracture

Diagnosis and Treatment of Stress Fractures

Early diagnosis of a stress fracture is important to prevent further injury. Your sports medicine physician will obtain a thorough history of the injury and determine the precise location by physical examination. Although X rays will usually be taken, in many cases a stress fracture will not show up in these films until healing has begun. As the fracture begins to heal, a bone callus will form that is usually visible on X ray three to five weeks after the injury occurs (Figure 10.2).

The most accurate method of diagnosing a stress fracture is with a bone scan, a specialized imaging technique that can detect small fractures in the bone within 48 hours after they occur (Figure 10.3). The earlier a stress fracture diagnosis is made, the sooner efforts can be taken to heal the injury and return you to full activity.

The treatment of an uncomplicated stress fracture involves modifying any activity that places stress on the injury, including running and jumping. Depending on the location of the fracture and the nature of your everyday activity, a cast is not usually necessary; however, a brace or rigid-soled shoe may be prescribed to keep the injured area immobilized.

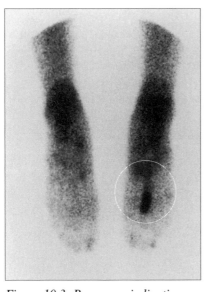

Figure 10.3: Bone scan indicating stress fracture

A stress fracture can take between six weeks and six months to heal completely, which is the amount of time needed for the bone to mend enough that reinjury does not occur. The average healing time is about eight weeks. During this period of healing, you can still keep fit by bicycling, swimming, running in a pool, and weight training.

Like other fractures, stress fractures can be slow to heal, a condition known as delayed union. This delay in healing can result from overactivity, metabolic conditions such as osteoporosis, anatomical considerations such as decreased circulation, or biomechanical factors. In these circumstance more aggressive treatment may be necessary, including cast immobilization, the use of external bone stimulation, or surgery.

When a stress fracture is the result of a biomechanical or structural abnormality, your sports medicine physician may also recommend orthotics, stretching, and strengthening exercises to reduce the risk of a repeat fracture.

If there are no contributing factors to your stress fracture, or if you suffer multiple stress fractures over a period of time, a thorough physical examination can determine whether a medical condition such as osteoporosis, an eating disorder, or a metabolic bone problem is contributing to the injury.

Stress fractures, which are a fear of most fitness-oriented individuals, usually heal uneventfully once properly diagnosed. Trying to run through this injury, however, is likely to prolong the healing process and possibly lead to more serious injury.

During a thorough examination, a sports medicine physician can help you identify factors that may have put you at risk for this injury as well as outline a plan of treatment to return you to full activity as soon as possible. ◢

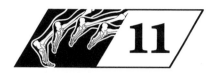

On Your Nerves
The Basics of Foot-Related
Nerve Injuries

ANYONE WHO HAS EXPERIENCED FOOT PAIN DURING FITNESS activities knows how much it can affect technique and performance. Foot pain can be caused by injuries to bones, ligaments, tendons, muscle, and other soft-tissue structures. It is also possible to injure one or more of the nerves that provide sensation to the foot.

When a nerve is injured, it usually results in paresthesia, which is an alteration in sensation, and may feel like pins and needles, numbness, or a sharp or burning pain. Very often, eliminating the cause of the irritation resolves these problems; however, if the irritation is left untreated, more serious problems can develop. The areas of the foot where active people most commonly experience these nerve problems are the toes, the inside of the ankle, and the top of the foot.

Morton's Neuroma
A neuroma is a thickening of a nerve that usually occurs from chronic irritation caused by tight-fitting shoes or socks, repeated pressure on the ball of the foot, or abnormal foot biomechanics such as overpronation that can result in injury to the nerve or its surrounding structures.

The most common location for a neuroma on the foot is between the third and fourth metatarsals and toes (Figure 11.1). Known as a Morton's neuroma, this condition usually has symptoms that include a burning or tingling sensation in the ball of the foot that radiates out to the third and fourth toes. You may also experience a cramping of the toes or a sensation that your socks are bunching up underneath your feet. If you remove your shoes and massage the area, these sensations will decrease, but the pain and discomfort usually recur when you resume activity.

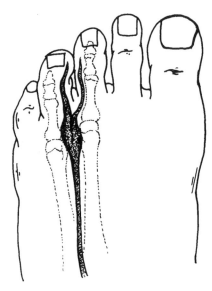

Figure 11.1: Morton's neuroma

Treatment for a Morton's neuroma involves removing the pressure that is causing the nerve irritation and reducing the inflammation around the nerve. Often, if you switch to an athletic or dress shoe with a wider toe box, the symptoms decrease or even disappear. Using a toe separator between the affected toes may also take pressure off the nerve.

If this self-care treatment does not relieve the discomfort, injection therapy can often reduce the inflammation around the nerve. If abnormal foot biomechanics are contributing to the problem, orthotics, combined with a metatarsal pad or other modifications to spread the metatarsals from each other, take pressure off the nerve. In most cases, conservative care will alleviate the problem. However, in resistant cases, it may be necessary to surgically remove the inflamed nerve branch to provide relief. This treatment will usually result in complete resolution of the problem.

Tarsal Tunnel Syndrome

People who use computer keyboards a lot are well aware of an injury in the hand and wrist known as carpal tunnel syndrome. A similar problem, tarsal tunnel syndrome, can occur in the foot. The tarsal tunnel is an area on the side of the ankle through which the posterior tibial nerve passes to enter the foot (Figure 11.2). This nerve branches off to supply sensation to the inside of the ankle and the bottom of the foot. If the tarsal tunnel becomes inflamed, it can constrict the nerve and cause the following: a burning pain along the inside of the ankle; a sharp, shooting pain that goes up or down the leg or foot known as

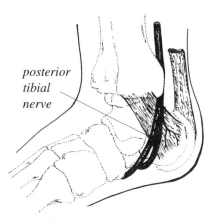

 is at the top left.

posterior tibial nerve

Figure 11.2: Posterior tibial nerve involved in tarsal tunnel syndrome

Tinel's sign; and even numbness along the bottom of the foot and heel. These symptoms can sometimes be confused with the pain of heel spur syndrome.

Tarsal tunnel syndrome can be caused by a direct or indirect injury to the nerve. It can also result from abnormal lower extremity biomechanics.

Once diagnosed, initial treatment for tarsal tunnel syndrome may include oral or injectable anti-inflammatory medication. Your doctor may also prescribe orthotics to control any abnormal foot or ankle motion that may be contributing to the problem. If the pain persists, your doctor may recommend a surgical procedure to release the structures impinging on the nerve. However, in many cases conservative care can resolve this problem if you treat it early.

Foot Numbness

Pain or numbness on the top (dorsum) of the foot is another common complaint of fitness-oriented people. Coursing along the top of the foot, very close to the skin, are small nerve branches that supply sensation to the top of the foot and toes. Because these nerves are so superficial, they are prone to irritation.

These nerves are usually injured by a shoe laced too tightly across the top of the foot or by prominent bones or bone spurs that cause irritation. The pressure from this irritation may lead to a pins and needles sensation or burning across the top of the foot. If left untreated, this irritation can progress to complete numbness in parts of the foot.

Initial treatment for this problem consists of loosening or altering the pattern of lacing your shoes to take pressure off the irritated areas on the top of the foot. You can also use moleskin or adhesive foam to pad any prominent bone spurs. Larger bone spurs may need to be removed surgically. However, if these bone spurs are the result of abnormal foot biomechanics, you can use an orthotic to slow the development of these prominences and in some cases eliminate the irritation to the affected nerve(s).

Many of these nerve injuries to the foot and ankle are due in part to temporary stresses that irritate the nerve. These problems can often be treated conservatively without a loss of training time. However, numbness, burning, and paresthesias can signify more involved problems, and you should be evaluated by a sports medicine physician if these symptoms persist. Seeking early evaluation and treatment may prevent the need for more involved treatment, and you will be able to resume your activities with pain-free feet. ◢

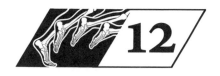

A Podiatrist's Perspective on Knee Injuries

THE KNEE IS A COMPLEX, HINGED JOINT THAT ALLOWS FLEXION AND extension of the leg and relies on a balance of the surrounding muscles, tendons, and ligaments to maintain stability during running and fitness activities.

The knee joint consists of the femur (thigh bone) and the tibia and fibula (leg bones), joined together by collateral ligaments on the outside and cruciate ligaments on the inside of the joint. Two C-shaped pieces of cartilage called menisci inside the knee help it absorb shock, and articular cartilage reduces friction and allows for smooth motion. The patella bone (kneecap) glides in a groove in the femur and helps protect the joint. Finally, tendons, which join muscles to bones, stabilize the knee. The quadricep muscles, in front of the thigh, help form the patella tendon that attaches the kneecap to the tibia.

Knee injuries may result from direct trauma or overuse. Direct trauma injuries usually come from direct blows in contact sports or from falls, jumps, sudden twisting, or explosive movements. Overuse knee injuries may result from overtraining, hard or uneven training surfaces, inappropriate or worn-out footwear, or structural or functional/biomechanical abnormalities of the lower extremity.

Structural knee problems may result from a misalignment of the leg due to inherited bone structure or because of a leg length difference. Functional/biomechanical knee problems can occur from a muscle imbalance around the joint or from abnormal foot or leg position or motion that causes the patella to move incorrectly on the femur.

Overpronation is the excessive rolling in of the foot that can occur during activity. Normal pronation makes the foot more flexible, allowing it to absorb shock as the foot hits the ground. As the foot pronates, the tibia rotates inward and the femur rotates outward. If the foot overpronates, this leg motion can cause the knee to be pushed out of alignment and stress the structures that surround and support it. Underpronation occurs when the foot does not roll in enough during the gait cycle and is often described as walking or running on the outside of your feet. This inadequate pronation can cause more stress on the outside of the knee, which can then result in overuse injuries to that area.

Traumatic knee injuries include tears of the collateral or cruciate ligaments, meniscus damage, or injury to the cartilage surfaces of the knee. These injuries are generally accompanied by pain at the time of the injury, swelling, and in some cases a locking or "giving way" of the knee. These types of injuries need prompt evaluation by an orthopedic physician to prevent the possibility of further damage to this joint.

Knee pain that develops gradually is often attributed to overuse or some form of biomechanical dysfunction of the lower leg. In the latter case, treatment must go beyond the injury to address the biomechanical factors contributing to its onset.

Common overuse knee injuries caused by structural or functional/biomechanical problems include patello-femoral pain syndrome (runner's knee), patella tendonitis, pes anserinus bursitis, popliteus tendonitis, and iliotibial band syndrome.

Patello-Femoral Pain Syndrome

Patello-femoral pain syndrome is one of the most common overuse knee problems in active individuals. Symptoms of this condition usually include pain around the front of the knee or underneath the kneecap. The pain is usually worse when you walk down stairs or run down hills and may also occur when you stand after sitting a long time with your knees flexed. The term chondromalacia patella is sometimes misused to describe nonspecific pain behind the knee. This latter term actually refers to a softening of the cartilage beneath the patella that can result from the same mechanisms as patello-femoral pain syndrome.

Patello-femoral pain syndrome can result from overtraining, weakness or muscular imbalance of the quadricep muscles, misalignment problems, and/or biomechanical abnormalities such as overpronation.

Treating patello-femoral pain syndrome often involves modifying your activity; icing for 15 minutes two to three times a day; judiciously using oral anti-inflammatories; decreasing activities like stair climbing, squatting, and running downhill; and correcting with orthotics any biomechanical problem such as overpronation.

Patella Tendonitis

Patella tendonitis or jumper's knee is commonly associated with fitness activities such as jumping and running that involve constant repetitive microtrauma. The patella tendon attaches the patella bone to the tibia (leg bone) in the front part of the leg (Figure 12.1). Symptoms of patella tendonitis can range from pain in this region after activity to pain with any type of motion in the knee. There may also be a small amount of swelling over the patella tendon. Usually the motion of the knee is normal.

Treating this condition usually involves appropriate stretches for the quadriceps and hamstrings, icing to reduce inflammation, activity modification, quadriceps strengthening, and patella tendon braces to keep stress off this area. If your doctor can identify biomechanical factors that are contributing to this injury, you may also benefit from orthotics.

Osgood Schlatter's Disease is often used to describe knee pain in adolescents that occurs in a similar location as patella tendonitis. Osgood Schlatter's Disease is an ir-

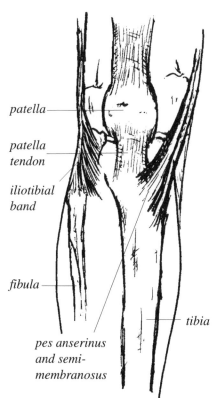

patella

patella tendon

iliotibial band

fibula

tibia

pes anserinus and semi-membranosus

Figure 12.1: Knee anatomy

ritation of the growth center at the top portion of the tibia bone and is aggravated by the same factors as patella tendonitis. There may also be a slight enlargement of the tibial tuberosity, a bone on the front part of the tibia. This condition is usually self-limiting and is treated conservatively in the same fashion as patella tendonitis.

Pes Anserinus Bursitis

Overuse knee pain occurring on the inside of the knee is often a result of overpronation that places stress in this area. This condition may be slightly more common in women because anatomical features such as wider hips can result in misalignment. The increased stress on this portion of the knee may irritate the ligamentous structures in this area, a group of tendons known as the pes anserinus that insert just below the knee (Figure 12.1). The pes anserinus consist of the tendons of the gracilis, semitendinosus, and sartorius. Underlying these cojoined tendons is a small, fluid-filled sac called a bursa that can also become inflamed as a result of a direct contusion or overuse.

The semimembranosus tendon, which is a part of the hamstring muscles, inserts on the medial side of the knee near the pes anserinus. A strain of this muscle can occur for similar reasons as a strain of the pes anserinus and can result in pain on the inside and back part of the knee.

The symptoms of these injuries are usually slow to develop but become more severe with activity. The pain can sometimes mimic that of meniscus damage.

Treating overuse medial knee pain includes modifying activity levels, ice, oral anti-inflammatories, and appropriate biomechanical control such as orthotics, if needed. If symptoms persist despite this conservative management, your knee may need further evaluation to determine whether a stress fracture, meniscal injury, hamstring tendonitis, or other condition is present.

Popliteus Tendonitis

Overuse pain in the back of the knee is often the result a popliteus muscle strain. This muscle helps the posterior cruciate ligament prevent forward motion of the thigh bone on the tibia during activity. Downhill running and overpronation put more strain on this muscle. The symptoms include pain on the outside back portion of the knee, particularly when you are running downhill.

PERRY H. JULIEN, DPM

Treating popliteus tendonitis includes activity modification, ice, oral nonsteroidal anti-inflammatories, and correcting any biomechanical asymmetries that may be present. You should avoid downhill walking or running while this injury is healing.

Iliotibial Band Syndrome

The iliotibial band is a fibrous structure that passes down the lateral (outside) aspect of the thigh and inserts into the lateral tibial condyle just below the outside of the knee (Figure 12.2). A small, fluid-filled sac called a bursa is located just underneath the iliotibial band at its insertion and helps reduce friction between the structure and the underlying bone. One of the functions of the iliotibial band is to provide stability to the lateral aspect of the knee during movement.

Tightness of the iliotibial band occurs when the distance between its origin and insertion is increased. This can be caused by such factors as overpronation, underpronation, or running on a crowned road. When this tightness occurs, flexion and extension of the knee during running activities produces an inflammatory response, as the tight iliotibial band rubs over the lateral femoral condyle. This condition is commonly called iliotibial band syndrome (ITBS).

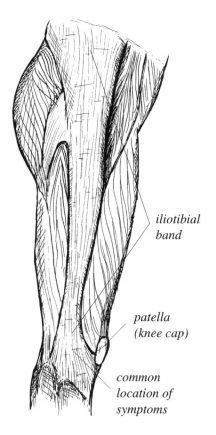

iliotibial band

patella (knee cap)

common location of symptoms

Figure 12.2: Iliotibial band

Runners and cyclists are more prone to ITBS-related knee pain because of the repeated knee flexion and extension that occurs during these sports. Increasing training distance or intensity can bring on ITBS, as can downhill running, lack of flexibility, running on a canted road, along with biomechanical abnormalities such as leg length differences, high-arched feet, or overpronation.

Symptoms of an iliotibial band injury include pain on the outside of the knee, especially when you flex the joint, walk down stairs, and run downhill. The knee may feel stiff, and if the bursa becomes inflamed, a small amount of swelling may be present. Your doctor will need to differentiate ITBS from other knee problems such as lateral collateral ligament sprains and injuries to the cartilage and other internal structures.

Initial treatment for ITBS involves determining what factors may have contributed to the onset of the injury. These factors must be addressed to prevent continued irritation of the iliotibial band. This may include altering your training program, changing running surfaces, and evaluating and replacing any worn-out shoe gear. Icing for 15 minutes several times a day and taking oral anti-inflammatories can reduce inflammation. Appropriate stretching of the lateral aspect of the thigh and sports massage therapy can also help provide relief for this injury.

If the pain persists despite these measures, your sports medicine physician may recommend physical therapy treatments such as ultrasound and a thorough biomechanical assessment to determine whether any structural or functional lower extremity problems are contributing to the ITBS. You may require orthotics if you have an abnormal biomechanical condition such as overpronation or underpronation. Likewise, if you have a significant leg length difference, you may need appropriate care for this as well. If the pain persists after a period of conservative management, your doctor may order further diagnostic tests such as magnetic resonance imaging (MRI) or bone scan to rule out other possible causes of the pain. In the most resistant cases, cortisone injections and even surgery may be required for relief.

You can often prevent ITBS with proper training techniques, including gradual increases in mileage and intensity, and shortening your stride when running downhill. Proper stretching and muscle balance can also reduce stress on the iliotibial band.

In addition, wearing the correct shoes for your foot type and activity and replacing them when they are worn-out will reduce undue force on the lower extremity during exercise. Finally, have your doctor identify and treat any structural or biomechanical abnormality that could lead to ITBS and other overuse injuries.

The first step in treating any overuse knee pain is self-evaluation and modifying the activity that might be causing the problem. This may include reassessing your current athletic shoes to ensure that they are appropriate for your foot biomechanics and replacing shoes that show significant wear. You should also reevaluate your training programs and training surfaces. Often overtraining or exercising on hard or uneven surfaces such as canted roads can contribute to overuse injuries of the lower extremity. If your knee pain persists despite these changes or is accompanied by increasing pain, swelling, locking, or giving way, you should seek an evaluation by an orthopedist. A thorough examination can determine whether or not more serious underlying problems are preventing your recovery. Often, conservative care consisting of protective taping or bracing, home exercises, and physical therapy can resolve these injuries. In some cases, surgery may be required if there is damage to the knee joint that does not respond to other forms of treatment.

When knee pain is not a result of trauma and its onset has occurred over time, or when no structural damage is found in the knee joint, the possibility exists that a biomechanical problem is contributing to this knee pain. In these circumstances, a podiatrist can be of help. Orthotics can often control biomechanical abnormalities such as leg length differences, overpronation, underpronation, and other lower-extremity asymmetries. These orthotics fit into athletic shoes and can control or correct misalignment problems of the lower extremity. Although orthotics are not indicated in all cases of knee pain, when used appropriately, they can treat overuse knee problems and prevent their recurrence.

Knee pain in active individuals can be the result of direct or indirect trauma or overuse. By establishing a correct diagnosis and determining the causes of the injury, the proper steps can be taken to return you to your fitness activities. ◢

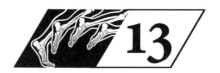

Orthotic Devices
A Biomechanical Approach to Treating and Preventing Injuries

ORTHOTICS ADD ANOTHER DIMENSION TO TREATING AND PREVENT-ing overuse injuries of the lower extremity. Despite their widespread use, there is still confusion about the types of orthotic devices available and their uses in sports medicine.

Most fitness-oriented individuals have used some type of foot-supporting device in their athletic shoes. Such devices range from sockliners that are built into the shoes and over-the-counter arch supports to orthotics prescribed by sports medicine professionals. Depending on the type of insert, these foot-supporting devices can increase comfort as well as prevent — and in the case of a prescribed orthotic, even treat — many types of lower extremity injuries.

Sockliner
A sockliner, or footbed, is the most common type of foot-supporting device and is considered part of an athletic shoe. Designed to make the foot more comfortable in the shoe, this type of insert generally absorbs a small amount of shock and has a small elevation to support the arch. In better-quality shoes, these sockliners are usually removable, which is useful if they need to be replaced by more precise arch supports or orthotic devices.

PERRY H. JULIEN, DPM

Arch Supports

Arch supports, available at athletic shoe and sporting good stores, are insoles that generally provide more cushioning and support than standard sockliners and are designed to replace them in athletic shoes. These arch supports are usually made from shock-absorbing materials and often have a small, built-in arch. Although arch supports do not control abnormal biomechanical motion, they do provide some foot support and protection against excessive shock to the lower extremity. One potential drawback is the generic rather than individualized placement of the elevated arch, which, if not compatible with the location of your arch, can cause some discomfort. Over-the-counter arch supports may also be helpful if you experience irritation, blisters, or pain resulting from bony prominences. Arch supports can also help treat mild cases of heel and arch pain (plantar fasciitis). However, in general, arch supports are designed more for comfort than for injury prevention and treatment.

Accommodative Orthotics

Another type of arch support is the custom footbed or accommodative orthotic. These are commonly called "soft orthotics" and are usually made from a mold taken while your foot is bearing weight. Soft orthotics generally provide adequate arch support but will not change or control any abnormal lower extremity motion. They are often used by individuals with high arches or those who need more support than is available with over-the-counter shoe inserts.

Functional Orthotics

Functional orthotics are foot-supporting devices that are usually prescribed by a sports medicine professional either to prevent or treat lower extremity injuries. A functional orthotic is a custom-made device that places the foot in a biomechanically correct position, allowing the muscles, tendons, ligaments, and bones to function more efficiently. These orthotics can be made from a variety of materials depending on the activities for which they are to be used and the problems they are correcting.

A functional orthotic consists of three components: shell, posting, and topcover (Figure 13.1). The shell is usually made from a thermoplastic material that is formed to molds taken of your feet, and it supports the arch in its neutral functional position. The mold from

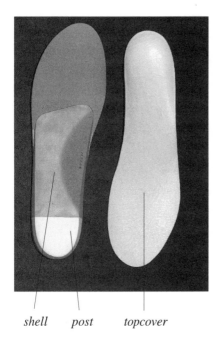

shell   post   topcover

Figure 13.1: Anatomy of a functional orthotic

which the shell is fabricated is usually made with plaster of paris applied while the foot is held in its corrected position. For most athletic orthotics, this is usually performed while you sit or lie without any weight on your feet. Your weight, foot type, and other factors determine the stiffness of the shell. Although rigid shells were initially used in athletic orthotics, it is now common for orthotics to be fabricated from a semiflexible material.

Posting involves using wedging to control and correct the biomechanical problems for which the orthotics are being prescribed. Posting may involve incorporating pieces of material on the bottom of the shell or modifying the shell itself. The topcover is placed over the shell to provide protection and shock absorption. In some instances, modifications can also be placed under the topcover to accommodate different foot types and biomechanical conditions.

Orthotics typically come in two lengths: three-quarter and full. The three-quarter length orthotic stops right at or just before the ball of the foot. This works well in dress shoes where bulk is a consideration. Figure 13.2 shows different types and sizes of orthotics.

Full-length orthotics are similar in size to the sockliners found in athletic shoes. This design enables you to remove the sockliner and replace it with the orthotic. By replacing the sockliner with the orthotic, you can prevent overcorrection, which may occur if you place the orthotic over an arch support.

Another advantage of a full-length orthotic is the capability of adding biomechanical correction or accommodation to the front part of the device. This is sometimes necessary in certain foot types or conditions and in runners who are midfoot or forefoot strikers.

Before you are prescribed orthotics, your physician will usually perform a biomechanical examination and a gait analysis. When you

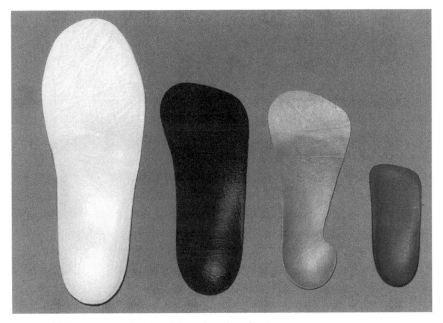

Figure 13.2: Types and sizes of functional orthotics

get your orthotics, there is a short adjustment period while your body adapts to the changes that have been made. In some instances, small modificatons may also be made to the orthotics to fine-tune them.

Biomechanics to the Rescue

The science of biomechanics has provided much of the framework from which orthotics have evolved. Lower extremity biomechanics involves the study of gait, foot stability, propulsion, muscle action, and how all of these relate to human motion. Although the perfect foot for a given sport or activity does not exist, there is a precise order of motion that must take place for normal foot function to occur. If something interferes with this motion, the foot and leg are forced to compensate for this deficiency, which may lead to pain or injury. Inflexibility, muscle weakness, ligament laxity, leg length differences, and inherited bone structure abnormalities can cause abnormal compensation to occur.

One of the most common ways the foot compensates is by overpronating. Pronation, the rolling in of the foot or the flattening of the arch that occurs normally when the heel strikes the ground, acts as the foot's own shock absorber to reduce stress to the rest of the body.

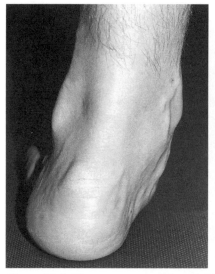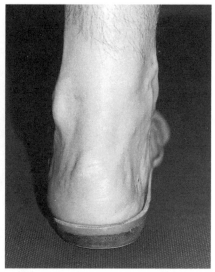

Figure 13.3: The overpronated foot (left) controlled with an orthotic (right)

After heel strike occurs, the foot needs to supinate or roll out slightly to convert the foot to a rigid structure from which to propel. However, if the foot needs to make up for motion unavailable elsewhere, it will continue to pronate, which results in an unstable foot. This foot instability can cause shin pain, plantar fasciitis, Achilles tendonitis, stress fractures, knee pain, and even bunions and hammertoes. Figure 13.3 shows how an orthotic can correct an overpronated foot.

How do you know if you need orthotics? Between 70 and 90 percent of all people have biomechanical imperfections, yet not all these people require orthotic control. Many fitness injuries are the result of overtraining, worn-out shoes, and other nonbiomechanical causes and can be treated without orthotics. However, certain foot types — an overpronated or high arched foot, for example — can be predisposed to overuse injuries. Since running activities place an impact of up to three times our body weight on the lower extremity with each stride, it is easy to see how even small biomechanical problems can become significant with increasing activity. In these situations, orthotics can control this abnormal motion, preventing an overuse injury from occurring. When an injury is already present, orthotics can place the foot in a more biomechanically correct position, allowing the injury to heal and preventing a recurrence.

Orthotics and Performance Enhancement

Performance enhancement through the use of functional orthotics is an area that requires more research. Although there is no proof that orthotics can make you run faster, they may indeed have a positive effect on your running activities by allowing your foot and leg to function more efficiently and by reducing the chance of injury.

Two sports in which specifically designed orthotics show some promise in increasing performance are alpine skiing and cycling. Orthotics designed for athletes in these sports reduce excessive motion and convert these movements directly to the ski or bicycle pedal with more efficiency. Modifications can also be made to ski orthotics to accommodate difficult boot fitting problems.

Biomechanical abnormalities can cause many overuse injuries that can become chronic if their cause is not addressed. While rest and other measures to reduce inflammation will relieve pain, your doctor should perform a biomechanical examination and gait analysis to determine if any structural or functional abnormalities exist that can be contributing to the injury. In these situations, a functional orthotic works by limiting or stopping the abnormal compensation and by providing shock absorption if needed, which allows the injury to heal and prevents a recurrence.

Footwear selection is also important in achieving maximum success from your orthotics. An orthotic controls the motion of the foot in the shoe, and the shoe must maintain this control when striking the ground. Shoe companies are continually designing sport shoes to provide increased motion control and shock absorption; your athletic shoe store can recommend shoe gear that complements the correction provided by your orthotics.

It is important to remember that orthotics prescribed for specific problems require an adjustment period to allow your body to adapt. When comfort is a prime concern, over-the-counter arch supports will usually suffice. However, for injury treatment or biomechanical control, functional orthotics can be an important part of the total treatment plan. They do not substitute for stretching and strengthening exercises, proper training techniques, and other treatments; however, when appropriate, orthotics can offer the injured and injury-prone individual hope of overcoming lower extremity problems. ◢

It's Not Always "Just an Ankle Sprain"

ANKLE SPRAINS ARE THE MOST COMMON ANKLE INJURY CAUSED BY fitness-related activities. Although ankle sprains are relatively common, they are often passed off as being "just a sprain" and thus not treated properly, which can result in long-standing pain, swelling, instability, and a limitation of your activities.

The ankle joint is formed by the two leg bones (tibia and fibula), the talus bone of the foot, a surrounding joint capsule, and ligaments on either side (Figure 14.1). The ligaments support the ankle joint. Most ankle sprains involve the ligaments on the outside (lateral side) of the ankle — the anterior talofibular ligament and the calcaneofibular ligament (Figure 14.2). Injuries involving ligaments are called sprains, in contrast to injuries involving muscles or tendons, which are categorized as strains.

Ankle Sprains

Ankle sprains most often result when your foot lands on an uneven surface, causing the foot to turn in as the ankle rolls out. This motion is called inversion and can result in a stretching or tearing of the ligaments and capsule on the outside of the ankle joint. At the time of injury you may hear or feel a pop or snap in the ankle and experience pain and difficulty while walking. Within a few hours the ankle may become swollen and bruised.

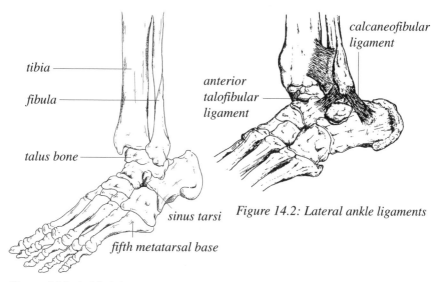

tibia

fibula

talus bone

anterior
talofibular
ligament

calcaneofibular
ligament

sinus tarsi

fifth metatarsal base

Figure 14.2: Lateral ankle ligaments

Figure 14.1: Ankle joint anatomy

Proper diagnosis and early treatment are important in the care of ankle sprains. Treatment should begin immediately after the injury occurs, even before you see a doctor. The sports medicine principle of RICE — rest, ice, compression, and elevation — applies to ankle sprains as well as other athletic injuries. The first step, rest, means you should get your weight off the injured leg to prevent further injury. Next, apply ice to the ankle. A good rule of thumb is to apply the ice for 15 to 20 minutes every two to three hours. Compress your ankle by wrapping it with an elastic wrap, and elevate it above the level of your heart to minimize the amount of swelling. RICE therapy will control the pain and swelling caused by the injury and facilitate a quicker recovery.

Ankle sprains are classified as first-, second-, or third-degree sprains, depending on their severity. A first-degree sprain usually involves a stretching of the anterior talofibular ligament. In a second-degree sprain the anterior talofibular and calcaneofibular ligament may be partially torn, and in a third-degree sprain there is usually a complete rupture of both these ligaments as well as the ankle joint capsule.

Seek medical attention as soon as possible after sustaining anything but a very minor ankle injury. Your doctor will want to take X rays of your foot and ankle to make sure you have not fractured any bones. Your doctor may also consider other diagnostic tests such as magnetic resonance imaging (MRI) to determine the extent of the ligament damage.

The treatment for ankle sprains depends on their severity. First-degree sprains may require that you take only a few days off while applying the RICE treatment. Second-degree sprains usually require immobilization with a brace to prevent further injury. Physical therapy and strengthening exercises may also be prescribed to speed your recovery. Third-degree ankle sprains may require you to have a cast and use crutches for several weeks. In the most severe cases, you may need surgery to reattach the torn ligaments.

Ligaments heal slowly, and after the initial period of immobilization, your doctor may instruct you on various exercises to decrease the likelihood that you will reinjure the ankle. In some circumstances a brace may be recommended for a period of time to provide additional support for your ankle during certain activities.

Recovery from an ankle sprain does not always require that you stop all athletic activities. Depending on the severity of the injury, your doctor can design an exercise program that will allow you to maintain fitness while your ankle heals. Riding a stationary bicycle or running in a pool with a flotation vest can provide an aerobic workout if you have a mild to moderate sprain, as long as you use a brace to prevent the ankle from turning in or out. You can also use selective weight training to maintain strength without compromising your recovery.

Ankle sprains that are improperly treated can result in long-standing pain and swelling, as well as instability of the ankle joint itself. The ligaments supporting the outside of the ankle are relatively small and are assisted in their task by two tendons known as the peroneus longus and peroneus brevis. When you don't allow a second-degree or third-degree ankle sprain to heal completely before resuming activity, the ligaments may lengthen. This lengthened condition can result in a loose joint that is prone to reinjury, especially when you participate in activities on uneven terrain.

Indicators of ankle instability include a history of repeated ankle sprains; pain, swelling or clicking in the joint during activity; and a sensation of weakness in the ankle. The best treatment for ankle instability is prevention, which involves aggressively treating anything more than a first-degree sprain with appropriate immobilization and rehabilitation to ensure full recovery.

If you have an unstable ankle, the first line of treatment usually involves using some type of brace or taping to prevent excessive motion at the joint. There are many types of braces available. However, their use is often limited by your ability to fit them into specific footwear.

Therapy is often used in conjunction with the bracing. This type of rehabilitation usually involves strengthening the peroneus longus and brevis muscles and tendons on the outside of the ankle and using specific exercises to improve balance and coordination. If you improve your sense of balance, your body will be able to respond more effectively to movements that could result in a reinjury of your ankle.

In some circumstances, abnormal foot biomechanics can predispose you to ankle sprains. In these cases, using orthotics can create a more stable platform for the foot and ankle and thus prevent recurrent sprains.

Although ligament sprains are recognized as the most common traumatic ankle injury, other problems can occur in this region as a result of twisting or turning the ankle joint. These problems include osteochondral fractures, fifth metatarsal fractures, and sinus tarsi syndrome. These conditions can often be mistaken for an ankle sprain and cause delays in proper treatment.

Osteochondral Fractures of the Talus

The talus bone of the foot and the tibia and fibula bones of the leg join to form the ankle joint. The articulating surfaces of these bones are covered with cartilage that provides a smooth surface for motion.

Any injury that places stress on the ankle joint can cause a defect in the cartilage. This can range from a slight compression or bruise to an actual fracture of the cartilage and underlying bone, which is known as an osteochondral fracture.

Symptoms of an osteochondral fracture can mimic those of a third-degree ankle sprain. In addition there may be pain on the opposite side of the joint from where the injury took place, or a clicking or grinding sensation when you move the joint.

Injuries to the cartilage surface of the ankle joint can often be hard to diagnose because cartilage itself does not show up on X ray. If an osteochondral injury is suspected, a CT scan or magnetic resonance imaging (MRI) may show more precise views of the cartilage and joint surfaces.

The initial treatment of an osteochondral fracture usually involves cast immobilization followed by therapy to rehabilitate the ankle joint. If the injury remains resistant to conservative care, your physician may recommend ankle arthroscopy, a procedure in which a small instrument is used to view the joint area and remove or repair any damaged cartilage.

Sinus Tarsi Syndrome

Although it does not involve an anatomical part of the ankle joint, sinus tarsi syndrome can often occur as a result of an ankle sprain. The sinus tarsi is a space on the outside of the foot between the talus and calcaneus (heel) bone (Figure 14.1). The sinus tarsi space is occupied by fatty tissue with small blood vessels and nerves running through it. Trauma such as an ankle sprain or an overuse injury occurring from repetitive stress can cause this area to become inflamed and produce pain just below the ankle joint on the lateral (outside) part of the foot.

Because of its close proximity to the ankle joint, sinus tarsi inflammation is often confused with ankle pain. However, closer examination will reveal that the discomfort is isolated to an area approximately one inch below the ankle joint. It may be accompanied by stiffness and decreased motion on the outside of the foot and ankle.

Initial treatment for sinus tarsi syndrome includes decreased activity and icing to reduce inflammation. If this approach is ineffective, one or two injections of corticosteroid into the sinus tarsi will usually provide relief. If there is an underlying biomechanical problem such as overpronation, your doctor may recommend orthotics to control any abnormal or excessive motion contributing to this condition.

Fifth Metatarsal Fractures

The peroneus brevis tendon is one of two tendons that provide stability to the outside of the ankle joint. The peroneus brevis inserts into the base of the fifth metatarsal bone on the outside of the foot. In severe inversion ankle injuries, the peroneus brevis may become taut and pull a small piece of bone off the fifth metatarsal (Figure 14.3). This is known as an avulsion fracture.

When this injury occurs, you will usually notice pain and swelling on the outside of the foot midway between the small toe and the back of the heel. X rays of the foot will usually confirm this fracture, and treatment involves cast immobilization until the bone is healed. This fracture can sometimes be slow to heal because of limited circulation in this area and the pulling effect of the peroneus brevis tendon on the bone as the fracture heals.

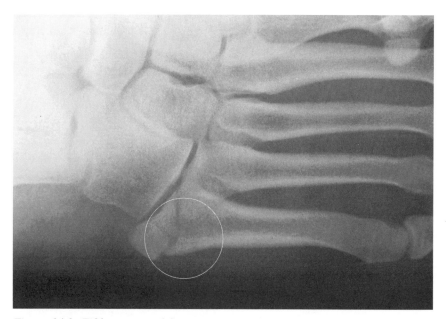

Figure 14.3: Fifth metatarsal fracture

Early diagnosis and aggressive treatment reduces the chances that ankle sprains and associated ankle injuries will linger or recur. Because ankle injuries are the result of a sudden trauma rather than overuse, they can be difficult to prevent. Wearing correct athletic shoes for your particular sport and being aware of obstacles and the surfaces on which you exercise can reduce the chance of injury. In addition, maintaining strength and flexibility in your lower leg can provide additional support for your ankle. Have your sports medicine physician evaluate any injury that causes swelling, significant pain, or a limitation of motion. The correct diagnosis and appropriate treatment will return you to full activity as soon as possible. ◢

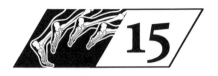

Toenail Troubles

TOENAIL INJURIES AND DISORDERS ARE COMMON IN FITNESS-ORIENTED individuals. Toenail problems can be caused by improperly fitting shoes, excessive perspiration, improper nail trimming, fungal infections, and congenital problems. This chapter looks at the causes and solutions of some of the more common toenail problems. Many of these problems do not require immediate treatment; however, a podiatrist should evaluate any painful condition that lasts longer than a week or becomes progressively worse.

Anatomy of a Toenail

The three components of the nail unit that are most often involved in toenail problems are the nail plate, nail bed, and nail matrix (Figure 15.1). The nail plate is what we commonly call the toenail, a structure made up of hardened skin-like cells that normally contain about 18 percent water. The softness or brittleness of the nail plate is due in part to how much water the nail plate contains.

The nail bed lies directly underneath the nail plate and contains blood vessels and nerves that make

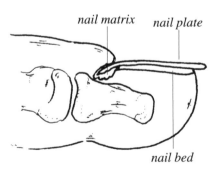

Figure 15.1: Anatomy of a toenail

PERRY H. JULIEN, DPM

this area very sensitive to injury. The nail bed also contains cells that help it adhere to the nail plate and contribute to the formation of the plate itself.

The matrix of the nail is located at the base or root of the nail and produces a majority of the cells responsible for forming the nail plate. The growth rate of a toenail is very slow and can take between 12 and 18 months for complete regrowth if a toenail is removed or falls off.

Black Toe

Black toe, also known as runner's toe or tennis toe, can occur in any sport, but runners seem to constitute a disproportionate number of sufferers. Black toe (Figure 15.2) occurs when the nail plate is either compressed or separated from the nail bed, causing blood to pool in the space between the two. At first the nail will appear reddish–blue, and after several days it will turn dark brown to black.

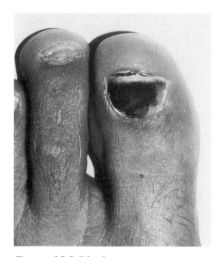

Figure 15.2 Black toe

If the discolored toe is not accompanied by pain, no treatment is necessary. The darkened nail will eventually either grow out or fall off, and in most cases it will grow back normal.

When the fluid build-up becomes excessive, the pressure may cause pain that can be relieved by draining the fluid that has gathered underneath the nail. Poke a small hole underneath the edge of the nail, as you would to drain a blister. Be sure to use a sterile needle, and keep the area clean to prevent infection. If the nail plate has not lifted, you may need to pierce the nail itself to reach this collection of blood and fluid. This procedure is best left to a podiatrist, who can use a small amount of local anesthesia to make this a painless procedure.

Once the fluid is drained, you should feel immediate relief, and you will probably be able to resume your normal activity within a day. In most cases the darkened part of the nail will eventually grow out. However, if the matrix or nail bed has been injured, the nail may remain detached or grow back deformed. Unfortunately, this condition is very difficult to prevent once the nail or its associated structures have been injured; if the pain or deformity is bothersome, you may wish to consult your podiatrist for treatment advice.

The best way to prevent black toe is to make certain your shoes fit correctly. When purchasing any type of athletic shoe, make sure that you have at least a ¼-inch of space between your longest toe and the end of the shoe. Also, be certain to try shoes on at the end of the day, wearing socks that you normally exercise in. Sock thickness and swelling of the feet both affect how well shoes fit.

Ingrown Toenails

The most common condition affecting the toenails is the ingrown nail. This problem occurs when the nail plate (usually of the big toe) presses into the skin on either side. If the nail breaks through the skin, an infection can result. The cause may be tight shoes or socks, incorrect nail trimming, or an inherited or acquired nail deformity. At first, you will notice pain and redness on the edges of the toenail. The surrounding tissue may then swell and sometimes leak fluid or pus. These symptoms usually indicate that an infection has set in that will usually require professional treatment for complete healing to take place.

Treating an ingrown toenail usually consists of removing the portion of the nail that is ingrown (Figure 15.3) and using foot soaks to resolve the infection. Your podiatrist may prescribe antibiotics in more severe cases. However, until the piece of ingrown nail is removed, the problem will usually not go away. Complications from an untreated ingrown toenail can include serious infection and ulceration. In most cases when treatment is initiated early, you can resume your full fitness activities within a few days.

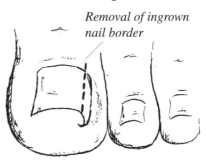

Removal of ingrown nail border

Figure 15.3: Treatment for ingrown toenail

You can prevent ingrown toenails by trimming the nail plate straight across, without leaving a sharp point in the corners. In addition, select shoes with a toe box that does not cramp your toes. If you frequently experience ingrown toenails, a podiatrist may be able to suggest ways to permanently remove the troublesome part of the nail.

Toenail Fungus

Infections caused by fungus are among the most frequent toenail problems and affect as many as 25 percent of individuals over age 30.

Fungal toenails are caused by organisms that thrive on the warm, dark, and moist environment of the foot inside a shoe. The chronic trauma that nails are subjected to during fitness activities can also predispose you to this problem.

Early signs of a fungal infection of the toenail include a gradual thickening and discoloration of the nail, which may become brittle and deformed (Figure 15.4), and may even disintegrate. Most of the time toenail fungus is not painful; however, in some cases the thickened nail can cause pain by pressing against the nail bed, hitting against the front of the shoe, or catching on socks.

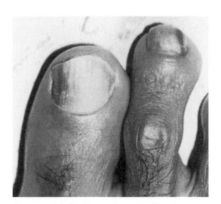

Figure 15.4: Fungal toenail

If you are not in pain, it is fine to do nothing about fungal toenails. Keeping your nails trimmed correctly and filing any thickened areas can reduce the chance of irritation, and over-the-counter or prescription topical antifungal medication may help resolve this infection over a long period of time.

If the nail becomes severely deformed or painful, removing the toenail is an option. This is not as traumatic as it sounds and can be done under local anesthesia in your doctor's office. In some cases the nail bed can then be treated with a topical antifungal medication. It is not uncommon for the nail to grow back deformed or for the fungus to recur, however, and in these cases a procedure called a matrixectomy can prevent the nail from ever growing back. Following this procedure, a hard, skin-like covering will form over the nail bed, which will allow pain-free fitness activity.

Some physicians prescribe oral medication to treat toenail fungus. These medications, although effective, can cause side effects, including liver complications and possible harmful interactions with other drugs. Most individuals should treat toenail fungus in a less aggressive fashion initially.

Subungual Exostosis

Subungual exostosis is a bone spur underneath the nail. Fortunately, it is not very common; however, it can cause considerable pain. The diagnosis of a subungual exostosis is made by taking an X ray. Usually, you will experience pain when you press straight down on the nail. This pain differs from the pain of an ingrown toenail, which in most cases will be painful on the sides of the nail plate. Conservative treatment for a subungual exostosis can include padding to relieve some of the pressure from the nail plate. However, in most cases, this is only moderately effective. The most definitive treatment is surgically removing the bone spur. This procedure can be performed under local anesthesia, and full recovery in most cases takes about a month.

The following recommendations should keep toenail troubles to a minimum:

- Trim your nails frequently, and do not leave any sharp edges at the corners.
- Use socks made from fibers that wick moisture away from the skin.
- Loosen your shoelaces when you're not wearing your shoes. This allows your shoes to air out.
- Pay careful attention to shoe fit, erring on the side of choosing a shoe slightly too large.
- Resist the urge to perform "bathroom surgery" on painful, infected, or deformed toenails. Instead, seek the advice of a podiatrist.

Toenail problems can be the source of much discomfort to the active individual. Many of the problems present only cosmetic concerns. When you have pain, however, seek appropriate treatment to prevent more serious problems from developing. ◢

First Aid for the Feet

MOST SPORTS AND FITNESS ACTIVITIES INVOLVE THE LOWER EXTREM-
ities. For this reason, even minor irritation to an area of the foot can
be painful. Many times, these small problems take a long time to heal
because of the constant friction to which they are subjected. The most
common foot complaints in this category include athlete's foot, ingrown toenails, blisters, corns and calluses, and warts.

Athlete's Foot

Athlete's foot (tinea pedis) is a skin infection caused by either fungus
or yeast organisms. The foot provides an excellent growing area for
these organisms because of the warm, dark, and moist environment
inside a shoe.

The symptoms of athlete's foot usually include itching, burning,
redness, and sometimes a dry, scaly appearance of the skin. This dry-
ness can result in skin cracking, which may allow bacteria to enter and
cause a secondary bacterial infection. A bacterial infection will usually cause warmth, redness, and pain on the surface of the foot.

To prevent athlete's foot, you must practice good foot hygiene.
Dry your feet thoroughly after bathing, and if possible, wear foot cov-
erings when using public showers and dressing areas. Use acrylic-blend
socks to wick moisture away from the foot, and consider using a foot
antiperspirant if you perspire excessively. You should also air out your
athletic shoes between usage; rotating between two or three pairs of

shoes will accomplish this. Regularly inspecting the skin between your toes and on the bottom of your feet will help you detect early signs of athlete's foot.

Athlete's foot can usually be treated with over-the-counter antifungal medications. Most of the symptoms should disappear after one or two weeks of treatment. If your symptoms last longer, or if pain and redness develop, see your podiatrist to make sure a bacterial infection is not present or to obtain a stronger, prescription-strength medication to treat the organism causing the problem.

Ingrown Toenails

Ingrown toenails commonly occur on the sides of the big toe but can affect any toe. Symptoms include pain and redness at the side of the nail. There may also be drainage coming from the nail border.

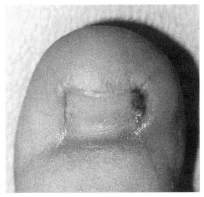

Figure 16.1: Ingrown toenail

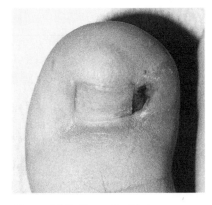

Figure 16.2: Toenail with ingrown portion removed

Ingrown toenails are caused when the nail plate presses into the skin around the toe and causes irritation (Figure 16.1). If the nail breaks through the skin, a painful infection may result.

Incorrectly trimming the nail is the most common cause of ingrown toenails. Toenails should be cut straight across to prevent the corners of the nail from cutting into the skin. Tight shoes and even tight socks can also cause the nail plate to be pushed into the skin. Some people have nail plates shaped in such a way that the nails become ingrown even with careful trimming.

Once a toenail becomes infected, it will usually not heal until the portion of nail causing the irritation is removed (Figure 16.2). Your doctor may recommend the permanent removal of the ingrown border to prevent this problem from recurring.

Although many people try home remedies and perform "bathroom surgery" for ingrown toenails, they should seek appropriate care from a specialist if the problem has not improved after a few days.

Blisters

Blisters result from friction on the skin that causes the skin layers to separate. This space then fills up with fluid or blood and forms what is called a blister.

Blisters are often caused by shoes that do not fit correctly or by pressure placed on a small area of the foot. Ensuring that your shoes fit correctly and have no areas of irritation from the tongue or stitching can help prevent blisters. Using acrylic-blend socks can also reduce the likelihood of blister formation because they reduce friction and wick moisture away from the foot. Vaseline or other blister-prevention ointments may be placed on pressure areas to reduce friction and decrease the incidence of blistering; however, some people are prone to blisters despite taking these precautions.

Treat a fluid- or blood-filled blister as follows:
1. Cleanse the skin with an antiseptic.
2. Using a sterile pin or needle, make one or two holes at the end of the blister and press on the side opposite the holes to force fluid out. Do not remove the skin on the top because it protects the healing area underneath.
3. Apply an antiseptic liquid or cream.
4. Cover the area with a protective bandage.

Most blisters should heal completely within a week. However, if you notice increased pain, redness, or drainage, you might have a bacterial infection, and you should consult with your physician.

Corns and Calluses

The medical term for corns and calluses is hyperkeratosis, which means "thickened skin." This skin thickening is usually the result of excessive friction on a part of the foot and is often attributed to shoe pressure over a bony prominence. Common areas for corns and calluses to occur are on the top of the toes and the balls of the feet.

Treating hyperkeratosis involves relieving pressure off the corn or callus, usually with moleskin or foam padding. You should never use medicated corn removers, as they have a tendency to burn or irritate the surrounding skin and can sometimes lead to an infection. Instead, reduce or remove the thickened skin by filing it away with a pumice stone or emery board.

If the corns and calluses persist, you may wish to seek advice from your podiatrist. In many instances, steps can be taken to lessen the pressure on or remove the bony prominences, which will reduce the formation of this thickened skin.

Warts (Verruca)

A wart, although usually appearing as an area of thickened skin, is actually a virus known as the papova virus. The term plantar wart refers to a wart occurring on the bottom of the foot.

A wart usually develops when the virus enters the skin through a small break or crack. This may occur from friction in an athletic shoe or some other minor skin trauma. The wart may develop within days or up to months after the virus enters the skin; in many instances, the virus remains dormant and doesn't cause any skin changes. Warts may be solitary or may occur in groups called a mosaic wart. The surface of the wart may have black specks resulting from superficial capillaries. Although some warts are referred to as being "deep", this is a misconception because a wart only grows to a certain layer of the underlying skin. However, this skin layer may differ in thickness depending on its location, which makes a wart appear to be deeper than it really is. Plantar warts, because they are on the bottom of the foot, are pushed inward into the surrounding, thickened skin.

Warts may or may not be painful, depending on their location. Because they are caused by a virus, they can spread, especially when the area is subject to the repeated irritation that occurs in athletic shoes.

Many people attempt self-treatment for a wart with various over-the-counter preparations that usually contain salicylic acid. Take care not to apply this wart medication to healthy skin, because it can irritate the tissue and in some cases cause an infection. If the wart remains resistant to treatment, enlarges, or increases in pain, your physician may recommend stronger medications or some form of surgical removal to resolve this problem.

Although skin and nail problems are typically not serious, any condition that causes pain in the foot has the potential to alter the way you walk, run, and exercise. This may place added stress on other parts of your lower extremities, resulting in other injuries that may be more difficult to treat than the initial problem. When self-treatment fails to alleviate any of these conditions or the problem worsens, a visit to your sports medicine physician may be appropriate. ◢◤

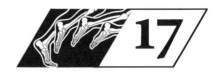

Leg Length Differences
The Long and Short of It

THE MOVEMENT OF THE LOWER EXTREMITIES DURING SPORTS AND fitness endeavors requires the coordinated efforts of muscles, tendons, ligaments, bones, and joints. An imbalance or asymmetry in any of these structures increases the likelihood that you will develop overuse injuries. This may result directly from too much stress being placed on specific structures or may occur indirectly as the body attempts to compensate for biomechanical imbalances.

Even though our lower extremities appear symmetrical, the left and right sides of our bodies are not always mirror images of each other. This asymmetry can be due to intrinsic factors relating to anatomy and biomechanics, or may be due to extrinsic situations such as worn-out footwear or uneven running and walking surfaces. One lower extremity asymmetry that receives a great deal of attention in sports medicine is leg length difference.

Types of Leg Length Differences
Leg length differences can be categorized as structural, functional, or environmental. Structural discrepancies result from an actual anatomic shortening of one or more of the bones of the lower extremity. This can occur from a growth plate injury during childhood or adolescence, fractures, or genetic and acquired conditions that affect bone growth. Structural leg length differences can also result from spinal abnormalities such as scoliosis.

Functional leg length differences usually occur as a result of muscular weakness or inflexibility at the pelvis or foot and ankle complex. The position of the pelvis can be affected by muscular imbalance, congenital bone irregularities in the pelvis or lower back, or improper posture when sitting or standing. Abnormal foot biomechanics such as overpronation in one foot or a significant arch-height difference between your two feet can also alter the functional position of the lower extremities even though the actual lengths of the bones are equal.

Environmental factors such as drainage crowns built into roadways, banked running surfaces, and even excessive wear of your shoes can create a situation mimicking a leg length difference. Additionally, these environmental factors can either accentuate or, alternatively, correct structural or functional length difference while you exercise on a given surface.

A leg length difference does not always produce symptoms. The body can sometimes compensate for these inequalities without causing significant alterations in biomechanical stress that could lead to injury. When a structural leg length difference is present, the foot on the long leg may pronate, effectively lowering the arch in an attempt to equalize the difference. The short leg may underpronate to further reduce this difference. If the foot on the long leg side overpronates more than is necessary to balance the structural difference, the longer leg may actually function as the shorter limb and result in a combined structural and functional lower leg discrepancy.

When the body cannot adequately compensate for leg length differences, symptoms ranging from foot pain to lower back conditions may develop. It is estimated that 60 to 95 percent of the population has some form of extremity asymmetry. Differences of up to ½ inch can often be compensated for during normal activity. However, ⅛-inch asymmetries can cause symptoms in active individuals due to the increased load and stress placed on the lower body.

Injuries caused by structural leg length differences tend to affect the long side first and include overuse knee pain, plantar fasciitis, shin pain, and metatarsalgia (pain on the ball of the foot). The short extremity may be predisposed to iliotibial band syndrome and injuries to the calf muscles and Achilles tendon. The symptoms on the long leg are often the result of compensations that are your body's attempts to functionally shorten the long limb.

Functional leg length differences tend to cause symptoms on the short side: overuse knee pain including iliotibial band syndrome, hip pain, plantar fasciitis, and shin pain. The most common symptom of both structural and functional leg length differences is back pain.

A leg length problem should be considered if an injury persists despite appropriate care. The exact measurement of a structural leg length difference can be difficult, but a good screening test is to lie on your back, placing your heels close to your buttocks with your ankle bones touching. If there is a height difference at your knees, a leg length difference may be present. Another way to screen for asymmetry is to stand in your shorts or underwear in front of a full length mirror and place your fingers on the top of your hip bones. If your fingers are not level with each other, a structural or functional leg asymmetry may exist. Finally, greater wear in the heel or ball area of the outersole of one shoe may indicate that the corresponding leg is longer than the other.

The treatment for leg length differences often depends on whether or not symptoms are present. If the body is compensating for a length difference without causing biomechanical stress in other areas, correcting the difference may alter your body mechanics in such a way as to cause an injury. If the discrepancy is causing symptoms, it needs to be addressed for full recovery to take place.

If your sports medicine specialist determines that your leg length difference is structural, treatment usually involves the use of either heel or full-sole lifts. Initially, your physician will usually utilize a lift equal to one half the anatomical discrepancy. This allows for a gradual realignment of the body structure and helps prevent the development of other injuries as a result of this correction. Generally, lifts up to ⅜ inch can be placed inside an athletic shoe. If more correction is required, an addition may need to be added to the outside of the shoe. The effectiveness of this form of treatment and the final amount of heel lift needed is usually assessed by feedback from the individual.

If you have a functional leg length inequality, your sports medicine physician needs to identify the underlying imbalance causing it. Once this is accomplished, treatment may include appropriate stretching or strengthening exercises, spinal or pelvic manipulation, heel lifts, or orthotics to correct biomechanical abnormalities of the lower extremity. If you have both structural and functional leg length differences, you may require a combination of these treatments.

If you develop symptoms consistent with a leg length difference, but a musculoskeletal examination does not reveal any asymmetry, you should make certain that factors such as uneven or banked training surfaces or worn-out shoes are not causing a situational or environmental leg length difference.

Although leg length differences are common, many active people with the condition never develop associated symptoms. However, when an overuse injury becomes resistant to treatment, you and your sports medicine physician should consider the possibility of a leg length difference. If an appropriate evaluation reveals a leg length difference, proper treatment for both the asymmetry and any injuries it caused will help you return to pain-free activity. ◢

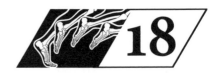

Surgery Is an Option
Common Foot Problems and their Surgical Treatment

THE FOOT IS A COMPLEX STRUCTURE REQUIRING THE COORDINATED function of 28 bones, approximately 20 muscles, and 112 ligaments to propel us in our everyday activities. Depending on the activities in which we participate, forces between one and three times our body weight are transmitted through our lower extremities with every step we take. It is no wonder that most people experience foot problems during their lives.

Despite their complexity and the stress constantly placed upon them, your feet should not be painful when you stand, walk, or participate in fitness activities. Pain, in most instances, makes us aware that something is not right.

Fitness-oriented individuals are reluctant to seek medical advice for their foot problems for fear that they will have to change their training habits. In fact, many problems, if diagnosed early, can be treated easily with shoe modifications, orthotics, exercises, stretching, and other conservative measures. When conservative therapy does not relieve these problems, or if pain becomes more severe, surgery may be suggested. Some of the more common foot problems that may require surgical treatment include bunions, hammertoes, and bone spurs.

Bunion (Hallux Valgus)

A bunion is an enlargement or bump on the outside of the big toe joint (Figure 18.1). Although usually considered a growth of bone, the bump actually represents a misalignment or partial dislocation of the first metatarsal phalangeal joint (first MPJ) (Figure 18.2).

Many factors can cause bunions. The most common of these is a muscular imbalance around the first MPJ. This imbalance can be caused by abnormal biomechanics such as overpronation or may be due to your specific foot structure. The latter explains why more than 30 percent of bunions run in families. Poorly fitting shoes by themselves usually do not cause bunions to develop, but they can accelerate or aggravate an existing problem by putting more stress on the area.

Bunions do not always cause pain, and in these instances, choosing shoes that have a wide toe box will reduce pressure on the area and decrease the likelihood of the bunion deformity becoming more symptomatic. Orthotics that fit into shoes can also help correct biomechanical abnormalities and thus eliminate some of the muscular imbalance that causes the toe to drift over.

Even when bunions become painful, the use of larger, wider shoes or orthotics may take enough stress off the inflamed area to relieve discomfort. However, as the angle in the big toe increases, friction from

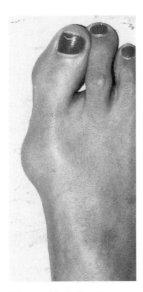 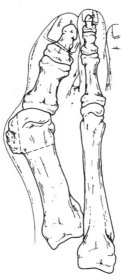 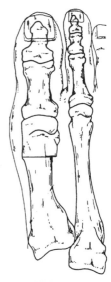

Figure 18.1: Bunion

Figure 18.2: Bunion showing misalignment of bones

Figure 18.3: Bunion after surgical correction

the joint angle will create further irritation and may cause enlargement of the first metatarsal head, making the deformity appear worse. When the pain or deformity progresses to the point that it limits activity and lifestyle, surgery may be necessary.

As the bunion deformity enlarges, the metatarsal bone is pushed out and widens the front part of the foot over time. This can damage the cartilage of the first MPJ and can also cause difficulty in shoe fitting.

In most cases, bunion surgery is performed to eliminate the pain caused by the deformity. Often, the pain is a result of pressure or irritation over the prominent bone, but it can also be caused by arthritis, which may develop as the toe drifts over. Bunion surgery, usually performed on an outpatient basis, involves removing the enlarged bump and realigning the joint (Figure 18.3). Once the joint is in alignment, there is less likelihood of the bunion recurring than if the bump is just shaved off.

There are many types of bunion surgery that can be performed, depending on your age, your activity level, and the severity of the deformity. Following a comprehensive evaluation and X ray, your physician will determine the most appropriate procedure for you. Most bunion surgery today involves removing a wedge of bone or making a cut through the bone in order to realign the joint properly. Once the joint is realigned, any excess bone on the side is shaved off.

The main concern of active individuals following any surgery is the amount of time that is necessary for recovery and return to full activity. This, of course, varies from person to person with bunion surgery, but generally individuals can participate in some type of cross-training activity such as swimming or riding a stationary bicycle after two weeks. These activities do not place undue stress on the surgical area while it is healing and can actually help reestablish range of motion at the joint. Full weight-bearing activities such as running, tennis, and aerobics must wait until the bone is fully healed, which can take from eight to twelve weeks. Following surgery, your doctor will in most instances recommend orthotics to control any abnormal biomechanical motion that contributed to the problem initially and to help prevent a recurrence of the bunion deformity.

Hammertoes and Corns

Hammertoes are another common bone deformity that can cause foot pain in active individuals. A hammertoe is a flexing or bending of one or both joints in a toe (Figure 18.4). The condition can be the result of inherited bone structure, muscle and tendon imbalance, or a biomechanical alteration in foot function.

As the toe becomes more flexed, it rubs against the shoe and causes irritation. Over time, the skin may thicken to protect the toe from this irritation. This thickened skin is known medically as hyperkeratosis and is commonly called a corn. Since a corn is the result of skin irritation from an underlying bone problem, corn removal medication provides no more than temporary relief for this condition and may actually damage the surrounding healthy tissue, possibly resulting in infection.

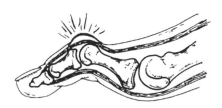

Figure 18.4: Hammertoe

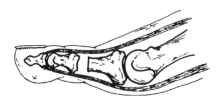

Figure 18.5: Surgical correction of hammertoe

When pain occurs from the bony prominences caused by hammertoes, early treatment may include using nonmedicated felt or foam pads to relieve pressure, selecting shoes with wider toe boxes, and using orthotics. Orthotics can be helpful in the early stages of a hammertoe, when the toe is still flexible and can be straightened by applying pressure underneath. In these situations, a metatarsal pad can be built into an orthotic to help align the toes correctly when the foot bears weight.

Over time, the angle of a hammertoe will become more rigid, making it impossible for the toe to straighten out. Constant pressure from shoes can create irritation, which may result in thickening of the bone on top of the toes. If the hammertoe has progressed so that conservative forms of treatment cannot relieve discomfort, surgery may be necessary.

Surgical treatment ranges from smoothing the enlarged bone to straightening the toe by removing a small piece of bone (Figure 18.5). The choice of procedure is based on the severity of the hammertoe.

Following surgery, patients usually can resume some fitness activities within a few weeks.

Once the bone spur is removed or the toe is straightened, the corn will usually disappear without additional treatment, because there is no longer any irritation to the overlying skin.

Bone Spurs

Although bunions and hammertoes are the most well-known bone deformities of the feet, other painful lumps and bumps can also form on parts of the feet as a result of chronic irritation.

These lumps and bumps, usually formations of extra bone, often result from abnormal biomechanical function of the foot or hereditary enlargements of certain bones. Although shoes are often blamed for these problems, they usually only aggravate an existing problem and therefore are only indirectly related to the discomfort.

Treatment for the bony enlargements depends upon their location, cause, and associated pain. Sometimes protective padding or changes in shoe model can relieve pressure. If a lump or bump results from a biomechanical abnormality, an orthotic may reduce the pain and prevent the problem from getting worse. When these measures are unsuccessful, surgery may be necessary to remove these bony enlargements.

Metatarsal–Cuneiform Exostosis

A metatarsal–cuneiform exostosis is a bone spur that occurs on top of the foot in the area of the instep. It often results from excessive motion in the joints caused by overpronation (flattening of the arch). The extra joint motion can jam the metatarsal–cuneiform joint, which may

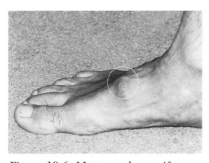

result in the formation of a bony lump on top of the foot (Figure 18.6). This bony enlargement can be further irritated by your shoes, especially where the shoelaces are. It can also cause numbness on the top of the foot due to compression of the small nerves that run through this area.

Figure 18.6: Metatarsal–cuneiform exotosis

Treatment for this problem consists of evaluating your shoes and possibly changing lacing patterns to take pressure off this area. If this is ineffective, foam padding can also reduce irritation.

Since a metatarsal–cuneiform exostosis is usually the result of a biomechanical problem, an orthotic with appropriate modifications can often reduce excessive motion in this area and can both relieve the pain and slow the progression of the deformity. If the enlargement remains painful, the bone spur can be removed, requiring several weeks away from sports activity. After surgery, your doctor may recommend orthotics to prevent a recurrence of this problem.

Enlarged Navicular

The navicular, a bone on the inside of the foot in the arch area (Figure 18.7), is one of the insertion points for the posterior tibial tendon, which resists overpronation. In some people, this bone grows dispro-

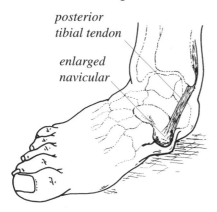

portionately large during adolescence. It can also grow in two separate pieces, which makes it appear larger.

When enlarged, this bone may be irritated by your shoes. Individuals with flat or overpronated feet tend to experience more pain with this problem because the posterior tibial tendon will become overstressed, causing inflammation.

Figure 18.7: Enlarged navicular

Initial treatment for this problem usually involves an orthotic to control overpronation and to relieve pressure from the inside of the arch area. If this is unsuccessful, surgery may be required to remove the portion of the bone that is enlarged.

Haglund's Deformity

A Haglund's deformity is a common bone spur on the outside of the back of the calcaneus (heel bone) near the Achilles tendon (Figure 18.8). Haglund's deformity usually results from irritation from shoes with hard or rigid counters such as women's shoes and ski boots. When a foot overpronates, the constant motion can also cause the bone in this area to thicken in response to the stress against the back of the shoe. A fluid-filled sac called a bursa may also form to act as a cushion. When this sac becomes irritated, it can cause bursitis in this area as well.

Early treatment for this condition usually involves padding to relieve the pressure and a heel lift to move the irritated area away from the shoe counter. Using cortisone injections is risky because the injury site is so close to the Achilles tendon. Orthotics may sometimes be effective in controlling abnormal motion in the shoe. If the Haglund's deformity remains painful, surgery may be indicated to remove the enlarged portion of the bone. Once the surgical area has healed you will often be able to return to activity after about eight weeks.

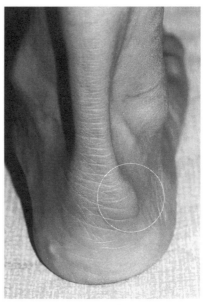

Figure 18.8: Haglund's deformity

Plantar Fasciitis/Heel Spur Syndrome

Heel spur syndrome is actually a misnomer. The pain experienced in this condition is a result of an injury to the plantar fascia, which is a band of tissue attaching to the heel and supporting the arch. Plantar fasciitis/heel spur syndrome is most often caused by repetitive stress at the junction of the plantar fascia and calcaneus (heel bone). This irritation results in pain. However, over time a bone spur may form as a result of this chronic irritation to the bone. The spur itself does not affect any of the surrounding structures and is in fact enclosed within the plantar fascia.

Most cases of plantar fasciitis/heel spur syndrome can be treated nonsurgically with measures to reduce inflammation and relieve the stress on the plantar fascia. The latter can be accomplished with appropriate stretches, arch supports, and orthotics when biomechanical irregularities of the lower extremity are noted. If conservative care over several months has not improved the symptoms and the pain alters your ability to exercise at the level you wish, surgical options are available for treatment.

Traditionally, surgery for plantar fasciitis/heel spur syndrome required a large open incision on the inside of the heel area to release the plantar fascia and remove the bone spur. This procedure often required a long recovery time.

More recently, a procedure called endoscopy has enabled a surgeon to release the plantar fascia without significant trauma to the surrounding tissue. This procedure, known as endoscopic plantar fasciotomy, is performed by placing two small incisions on each side of the heel into which an endoscope, or small camera, is inserted. The endoscope allows the surgeon to see the plantar fascia, which is then released using a special instrument. The heel spur itself is not removed, as this is not usually a cause of the symptoms. Following the procedure, immediate weight bearing is usually allowed.

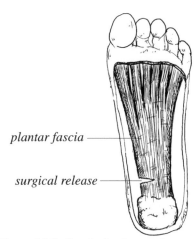

plantar fascia

surgical release

Figure 18.9: Surgical release of plantar fascia

However, it may still take several weeks for full healing to take place, and during that time weight-bearing activity should be restricted. Despite the shortened recovery period for this procedure, you should consider plantar fasciitis/heel spur syndrome surgery only after you have exhausted your conservative treatment options.

Many treatment options are available for these foot complaints, and, if they are identified early, your doctor may be able to offer you conservative treatment not only to eliminate pain but also to prevent the problem from getting worse. However, if your condition has progressed to the point that conservative treatment does not relieve your discomfort, then surgery may be recommended.

Foot surgery can be effective in both relieving pain and correcting deformities. Although a recovery period is necessary, your doctor may allow activity such as stationary bicycling, swimming, or running in a pool once adequate healing has begun. This short time away from your normal activity is usually a small sacrifice compared to the limits that the constant discomfort of untreated foot problems can place on you. ◢

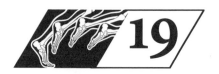

Little Feet
A Primer on Children's Foot Problems

CHILDREN'S SPORTS AND FITNESS INJURIES CAN DIFFER FROM THOSE of adults because of the immaturity of young bones, ligaments, muscles, and tendons. Frequently, these injuries are passed off and ignored as "growing pains." However, certain overuse injuries left untreated in a young, active person can result in further complications as the child grows older.

Growth Plate Injuries

When children complain of lower extremity pain in joint areas, it is important to evaluate the growth plates located in the bones of the feet and legs (Figure 19.1). The growth plate, or epiphysis, is an area at the end of the bone that produces bone tissue to allow for growth. These growth centers normally begin to close at age 15 in boys and age 13 in girls. These growth centers may not close completely until age 18, depending on the growth center of the specific

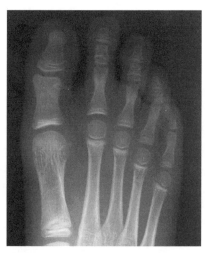

Figure 19.1: Open metatarsal growth plates

PERRY H. JULIEN, DPM

bone. Any injury that cases damage to the growth center can alter the growth of that bone.

There are two ways that growth centers can be injured: by a sudden direct force, such as a sprain or fracture, or by overuse. Bones are connected to each other by ligaments. A child's developing bones are often weaker than their ligaments, which makes it more common for a child who suffers a direct injury to fracture the bone or disrupt the growth plate than to tear a ligament. In an adult, a ligament will usually tear before its connecting bone becomes fractured.

Any twist or fall that results in pain or swelling around the joint in the foot or leg should be properly evaluated by a sports medicine physician. In most instances, X rays will be taken of the injured area, as well as the opposite leg or foot, to make certain that the growth plate has not been damaged. If an injury to the growth plate has occurred, it must be treated right away to prevent any damage or deformity in the growing bone.

Osgood Schlatter's Disease (Jumper's Knee)

Osgood Schlatter's Disease, which usually occurs in active children between the ages of 10 and 15, is most often caused by an overpull of the patella tendon that joins the thigh muscles to the kneecap. Constant stress on this area from running or jumping will result in an inflammation of the growth plate on the top part of the tibia (leg bone). The injury is very common in basketball, soccer, and running sports. Symptoms of Osgood Schlatter's Disease usually include local pain and tenderness with some mild to moderate swelling. The child may also limp and have difficulty climbing stairs. This injury is caused by the same forces that will result in patella (kneecap) tendonitis in an adult. A thorough evaluation will usually rule out the presence of other problems that can also occur in this area.

Modifying the child's activity and using ice therapy are the initial treatments for this injury. Your sports medicine physician may also recommend appropriate exercises to improve the child's flexibility and strength around the injured area. If there are biomechanical imbalances such as overpronation, the doctor may recommend orthotics. Osgood Schlatter's Disease can be short-lived or may cause frequent pain until the growth plate closes. The symptoms usually resolve completely at that time; however, a small knot of bone that is usually not painful may remain as a result of the previous irritation to this area.

Calcaneal Apophysitis

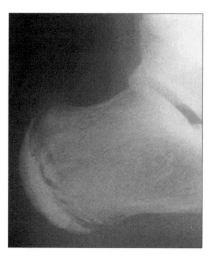

Figure 19.2: Growth plate (calcaneal apophysis)

Calcaneal apophysitis, or Sever's Disease, is the most common cause of heel pain in children between the ages of 8 and 16. The calcaneal apophysis is the growth plate located on the back of the heel bone (calcaneus) (Figure 19.2). Both the Achilles tendon and plantar fascia insert into this area and exert a pulling stress on this growth plate. In addition, the constant pressure on the heel caused by running or jumping can irritate the growth plate.

Symptoms of calcaneal apophysitis are usually present during activity and are located in the back or bottom of the heel. The heel may be painful if it is squeezed from the sides. Walking, running, and other forms of weight-bearing exercise seem to aggravate this problem. There is usually no swelling, and the child may not recall any single episode that caused the pain.

Early evaluation is necessary to rule out other causes of heel pain in children, including fractures of the heel bone, penetrating objects such as thorns or shards of glass, and infection.

Initial treatment for calcaneal apophysitis usually involves using heel lifts to take pressure off the tendons and fascia that pull on this area. The heel lifts also cushion the heel. A biomechanical evaluation may reveal abnormalities such as overpronation, which can also contribute to this condition and can often be corrected with appropriate stretching or orthotics.

In many cases, the child can continue with activities on a reduced level until healing is complete. If the pain alters the child's foot strike, the child may need to rest the foot completely. Very rarely is cast immobilization necessary. As with other growth plate irritations, calcaneal apophysitis will resolve completely once the growth plate has closed, usually around age 16. If the onset of calcaneal apophysitis is due to biomechanical abnormalities in the lower extremities such as overpronation, the mechanisms that led to this condition could result in plantar fasciitis or heel spur syndrome in adulthood.

PERRY H. JULIEN, DPM

Stress Fractures

Lower extremity stress fractures usually result from repetitive microtrauma in sports that involve running and jumping. A stress fracture occurs when the bone fatigues to the point that it develops a fracture. Stress fractures are usually not associated with a single traumatic episode and can sometimes be difficult to diagnosis by X ray because the bone generally stays in good alignment after fracturing.

A young athlete with a history of eating disorders such as anorexia or bulimia is more likely to develop stress fractures. These disorders compromise the normal nutritional requirements in active individuals and can lead to bone weakening. Overtraining, especially on hard surfaces, can also increase the risks of developing stress fractures.

The treatment for a stress fracture usually involves stopping weight-bearing exercise for 6 to 12 weeks. It is also important that the doctor identify any factors that may have led to the injury and correct or modify these as appropriate.

Biomechanical Foot Abnormalities

A wide range of foot types are considered normal in young children; however, severely flat feet or high-arched feet may indicate a problem that can lead to injury. Pronation is the rolling inward of the foot (flattening of the arch) that occurs normally to help reduce impact when the heel hits the ground. However, overpronation can affect normal foot function and predispose a young athlete to problems in the lower extremities (Figure 19.3). Overpronation can be hereditary or result from tight calf muscles, leg length differences, bow legs, or imbalances within the foot. If left untreated, overpronation can lead to painful flat feet, bunions, and overuse injuries. It is also possible in certain cases for knee, hip, and back pain to be related to poor foot function.

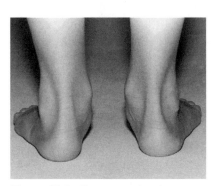

Figure 19.3: Overpronation in an eight-year-old child

The treatment for overpronation ranges from exercises and shoe modifications to orthotics, depending on the severity of the deformity and any symptoms present. Early intervention in cases of severe overpronation can often prevent the development of more significant problems as the child grows.

Children with rigid, high-arched feet are not able to absorb impact very well, which can result in stress-type injuries to the foot and leg. High-arched feet may be inherited or in some cases result from certain diseases. A thorough lower extremity examination can determine whether treatment is necessary. Often, careful shoe selection and, when necessary, orthotics can help prevent problems due to this foot type.

Proper Shoe Selection

Selecting proper athletic shoes is as important in preventing injuries in young athletes as it is in older athletes. Today, most athletic shoes are designed for specific sports such as tennis or running. The components that go into making these shoes provide protection during various motions that occur in different sports. It is important to select a shoe that not only fits well but also is appropriate for your child's foot type and activities. A sports medicine podiatrist, along with a shoe-fitting specialist, can help determine the best type of shoe for each child.

Sports and exercise can be a vital part of a child's health plan. The same precautions that adults should take prior to participating in any health and fitness activity apply to children as well. These precautions include developing a good warm-up and cool-down routine, maintaining adequate lower extremity flexibility, and learning correct technique for the activities in which they are participating. When injuries do occur, whether they result from trauma or overuse, early evaluation and treatment very often allow children to continue participating in the activities they enjoy without running the risk of further injuries. ◢▰